Your Foundation in Health and Social Care

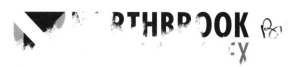

Your Foundation in Health and Social Care

A guide for Foundation Degree students

Edited by
Graham Brotherton and Steven Parker

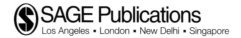

SAGE Publications
Los Angeles • London • New Delhi • Singapore

SAGE Publications Ltd
1 Oliver's Yard
55 City Road
London EC1Y 1SP

SAGE Publications Inc.
2455 Teller Road
Thousand Oaks, California 91320

SAGE Publications India Pvt Ltd
B 1/I 1 Mohan Cooperative Industrial Area
Mathura Road
New Delhi 110 044

SAGE Publications Asia-Pacific Pte Ltd
33 Pekin Street #02-01
Far East Square
Singapore 048763

Library of Congress Control Number: 2007929031

British Library Cataloguing in Publication data

A catalogue record for this book is available from the British Library

ISBN 978-1-4129-2039-1
ISBN 978-1-4129-2040-7 (pbk)

Typeset by C&M Digitals (P) Ltd, Chennai, India
Printed in Great Britain by The Cromwell Press Ltd, Trowbridge, Wiltshire
Printed on paper from sustainable resources

CONTENTS

NOTES ON CONTRIBUTORS

Ruth Beretta is a Curriculum Area Manager and Lecturer in Social Sciences, Social Work and Health Professions at Cornwall College, Camborne. Her background is in nursing and nurse education having come to Cornwall from Coventry University. Her areas of interest are in the experience of students in higher education and the development of transferable skills through education and public policy.

Graham Brotherton is a Senior Lecturer in Policy Studies at Newman College of Higher Education in Birmingham with a particular interest in teaching and researching children and family policy. He has taught in both further and higher education institutions and has been actively involved in the development of Foundation Degrees. In a previous career he was a worker and manager in a range of health and social care settings.

Judith Mann is a Lecturer and Programme Manager at Cornwall College, Camborne. Her first career was in social work, with a particular interest in mental health and children and family work. She currently teaches on both a Foundation Degree (Health and Community Studies) and a Social Work degree.

Robert Mears studied at Leicester and London Universities and has taught undergraduates and health professionals at Leicester University, the Open University and University College Northampton. He joined Bath Spa University in the early 1990s where he is currently Professor of Sociology and Head of the School of Social Sciences. He teaches on Sociology and Health Studies courses and supervises Masters and research students in Sociology and Health Studies.

Steven Parker is a Lecturer at Somerset College, Taunton, where he manages the higher education provision within the Division of Social and Professional Studies. He is also an Associate Lecturer with the Open University and has worked as a social worker in the voluntary and statutory services.

Nadine Pearce is a Lecturer and Programme Manager for the FdA Health and Community Studies in the Department of Social Sciences, Social Work and Health Professions at Cornwall College, Camborne. Her background is in nursing and nurse education and she currently teaches psychology modules on a range of programmes including Foundation Degrees in Health and Community Studies, Complementary Health Therapies, Healthcare Practice and on the CFP for Pre-Registration Nursing.

INTRODUCTION

Welcome to *Your Foundation in Health and Social Care*. This book has been written to support students taking Foundation Degrees, and all of the contributors have some experience of Foundation Degrees in Health and Social Care. It is hoped that it will also be useful to students on related higher education courses. It could also support NVQs at Levels 3 and 4. The book is designed to support you in at least three ways:

- By providing you with advice on different aspects of your programme, e.g. academic study skills or making the most of placement/work-related learning.
- By providing you with chapters dealing with key areas of study you are likely to encounter on your course.
- By identifying useful sources of additional information to support you in your studies.

In order to do this the book is divided into two sections together with a final chapter which pulls together the themes of the book. The first section consists of Chapters 1–3 and looks at approaches to studying. Chapter 1 focuses on study skills and how to approach the academic part of your course. Chapter 2 looks at getting the most out of placements and work-related learning and Chapter 3 looks at identifying research and information to support your course and at how to evaluate the usefulness of different sources of information.

In the second section (Chapters 4–9) there is an overview of a range of areas relevant to studying health and social care. Chapter 4 considers the social context, Chapter 5 the role of values and ethics and Chapter 6 the organisational context. Chapter 7 deals with psychology for health and social care, Chapter 8 with interpersonal skills and Chapter 9 with assessment and care management. The final chapter seeks to pull together some of the key themes of the book and look at where health and care services might be going.

Health and social care has undergone a dramatic period of change over the past 20 years and this shows no signs of abating. Whether you work in the health sector or adult or children's social care, both the structure of services and ideas about what constitute good practice have changed considerably and it is already clear that this process is going to continue. Words like empowerment advocacy and concepts like consumerism and the mixed economy of care (all of which are explored in this book) are forcing us to look carefully at almost everything we do. You are therefore either entering or developing your career at an interesting and challenging time. The challenges of working in a vital area of work at a time when the population is both ageing and becoming more diverse will create a new range of both opportunities and problems and will require us all to rethink many areas of policy and practice in ways that will affect the whole workforce. Issues such as how we decide who gets access to services, under what circumstances, how much 'say' they have about the services provided for them, and who provides the services in the first place, are all central and at times controversial issues discussed throughout the book. These are questions on which there are differing perspectives and about which you need to think carefully from your personal perspective. We hope the book will help you in thinking about these issues as your course progresses.

How to use this book

This book is intended to give you an overview in relation to each of the areas it covers. As the courses it supports are higher education courses, it cannot and should not be the only source you use and while we aim to give a clear overview for each topic you will need to read/research more fully. To help with this each chapter has suggestions for further reading and Chapter 3 contains detailed advice on where you can look for appropriate material to support your studies.

It is hoped that this book will support you throughout the duration of your course and that you will 'dip' in and out of the material throughout your studies. Within each chapter there are a range of activities designed to help you to think about key ideas and issues and it is hoped that you will pause and reflect on these as the opportunity to reflect is an essential element of learning. Some chapters also includes some final questions; again these are to help you to reflect upon and apply the chapter's content.

Using the language of health and social care

In coming to terms with completing a course in higher education it is important to learn the professional language of health and social care. While every effort has been made to avoid jargon, there are inevitably terms with which you will not be familiar. These are explained within the text; however, if terms either within the text or in your wider reading are not familiar to you there is an excellent and very comprehensive glossary of health and social care terms available at the http://www.cpa.org.uk web site.

In concluding this brief introduction we would like to take the opportunity to wish you every success with your studies and hope that this book contributes to successful completion of your studies.

SECTION ONE

Approaches

1 APPROACHING LEARNING

Ruth Beretta

SUMMARY CHAPTER CONTENTS

- Learning in higher education
- Learning how to learn
- Learning styles
- Managing time effectively
- Effective reading and note taking
- Writing essays and reports
- Using references and bibliographies
- Plagiarism and how to avoid it

Learning objectives

By the end of this chapter, you should be able to:

- Identify some of the challenges in successful study in higher education and how you can work to overcome these.

- Identify your preferred learning style and adapt learning strategies to help you make good use of your time and develop your learning skills.

- Use effective reading and note-taking skills.

- Make good use of reading lists and assignment guidelines to produce constructive essays and reports.

- Reference academic writing with a recognised referencing system and avoid plagiarism.

Introduction – learning in higher education

In this chapter we will be focusing on how to study in higher education. We have assumed that you are new to higher education study, but even if you are not you may find it helpful to refer to this chapter to remind yourself of some of the key issues around studying at this level. A Foundation Degree has a slightly different emphasis to other degrees because it explicitly integrates academic and work-based learning. It emphasises the importance of working in your chosen profession in the area of health and social care as well as studying at a higher level at college or university.

However, learning in higher education by itself can be quite a challenge and you may need to prepare yourself for a different way of learning.

Learning *how* to learn

When working as well as studying on a course, many of us need to make best use of our time and ensure we develop our skills and knowledge base as effectively as possible. For many people, that means learning *how* to learn. It sounds very straightforward, but often we have memories of time spent at school, which may have been a negative experience. However, we all have the capacity to develop study skills which can improve our time management and make for effective academic skills.

Why are you doing this course?

It may be useful to spend a few moments reflecting on your own motivation for starting the Foundation Degree programme and considering:

- Why am I doing this course?
- What knowledge and skills do I already have?
- What knowledge and skills do I hope to gain?
- What has previously helped me to make opportunities for study?
- What may get in my way?
- How can I ensure I have the best possible chance of success?

Obviously, the answers to these questions will be personal and depend upon your own circumstances. But if you can think ahead to find answers to these questions, you will be better prepared to meet the challenges you may face as your course progresses. This is why learning how to learn is so important.

One other reason is that there is an expectation that, as a graduate, you will have developed a wide range of skills, experiences and qualities during your course, as well as gaining a broad knowledge base. These skills and qualities, are shown in the box below.

Graduate skills and qualities (from Cottrell, 2003)

1 Traditional skills associated with knowledge

Ability to:

- Organise, summarise and analyse material
- Make sense of complex information
- Make critical selection and evaluation of evidence
- Argue logically and apply theory to practice
- Challenge taken-for-granted assumptions
- Study a subject in depth and breadth
- Demonstrate subject specific skills, including technical skills

2 Key skills

Including:

- Communication
- Application of number
- Information and communications technology
- Improving one's own performance, including study skills, personal development planning, self-direction and self-evaluation
- Working with others
- Problem solving

3 Personal qualities

Including:

- Self-reliance and independence
- Adaptability, flexibility and openness to change
- Ability to take responsibility
- Creativity and imagination
- Ethical awareness

4 Preparedness for work

Including:

- The skills identified above
- Career planning
- Understanding how organisations work
- Ability to work effectively
- Skills related to a chosen area

In thinking about the challenges ahead, you may well see managing your time effectively as a key area, especially as you are likely to be working as well as studying for your course. You also need to be aware (if you are not already) that learning in higher education is likely to be different to the study you undertook at school. Some of those differences include the use of time and the approaches adopted towards learning:

- Use of time:
    - (a) You have much more flexibility in how to use your time. If you decide not to attend lectures, you may not be asked to account for where you have been, so it is up to you how you spend that time.
    - (b) You will be given assignments at the beginning of term which should be produced by a given deadline; you may not be given further prompts about the work, so you need to be organised.
    - (c) There is an expectation that you will use time away from college or university to read extensively around your topic area.
- Approaches towards learning:
    - (a) You are given responsibility for your own learning and it may be up to you to seek tutorial support rather than a lecturer asking to see you at regular intervals throughout the course.
    - (b) Learning in higher education is not just remembering facts: it is about using or applying those facts and evaluating them.
    - (c) You may find yourself allocated to large groups for key lectures where you know very few other students, which can be frightening.
    - (d) Members of teaching staff are known as lecturers rather than teachers and you may need to make an appointment in order to see them.
    - (e) You will be expected to read your course handbook and be aware of issues such as regulations regarding handing in work, referencing styles and procedures governing your course.
    - (f) You can expect a wide range of learning and teaching methods to be used, as well as academic jargon you may not be used to.

See also Table 1.1.

Learning styles

We all learn things in different ways and it is important for you to recognise what works best for you.

Activity

How do you learn best?
Think back to an experience when you found it very easy or very enjoyable to learn something. It may have been a household project, something at work

or even an experience from school. What was it that made it a good learning experience? Was it the teacher? Was it because you were particularly interested in the topic? Was it the way you were taught?

Now think back to a learning experience that was difficult or unpleasant. What happened that was different to the first experience? Do you think the situation could have been managed differently?

What do these experiences tell you about the way you learn best?

You may have identified that you enjoy learning experiences which actually involve physically doing something. It is much easier to learn how to bake a cake by mixing the ingredients together and watching the mixture satisfactorily rise in the oven than just to read a series of recipes! And having a conversation with a hearing-impaired person teaches you much more about communication skills than any textbook!

You may associate a poor learning experience with an impatient teacher who does not like to be interrupted by questions, or with a period of inactivity. For some topics such as human biology, there is no substitute for learning about body organs and systems to understand how the body works by studying anatomy texts. But it becomes much more interesting when that knowledge is used to inform us about how medications work in the body, or how disease processes attack the body.

On the other hand, you may have associated a good learning experience with a lecture in which you gleaned a great deal by listening to an expert talking about his or her topic area with enthusiasm and then being stimulated to read up on the topic following the lecture. You may have considered a poor experience to be an unstructured session when you were preparing groupwork for a later presentation.

This shows us that there are a number of learning styles and we respond differently to different situations. It has been suggested that we should identify which is our preferred learning style and aim to use this style as often as possible to maximise our learning. One (of many) ways of looking at this is the VARK model.

VARK categories

These are categories of learning styles which we may use:

Visual (V):

This preference means you prefer to use visual information for learning, such as charts, graphs, diagrams.

Aural/Auditory (A):

This means you prefer to learn by hearing material such as lectures, group discussions, presentations and tutorials.

Read/write (R):

This means you prefer to learn by seeing information displayed as words, so you prefer to read and make notes.

Kinaesthetic (K):

This means you prefer to learn by movement or by actually doing something, so you would prefer to learn 'on the job' or by role play, or by a mixture of activities in a session.

TABLE 1.1   *LEARNING AND TEACHING METHODS IN HIGHER EDUCATION*

Lecture	Traditionally used to address large numbers of students, often in a lecture theatre with raked seating. Usually, the lecturer speaks directly to the students while they take notes. There is usually little interaction between the lecturer and students
Seminar	A seminar gives the opportunity to meet in smaller groups and the focus of the seminar may be a recent lecture or some pre-set reading. A seminar should encourage participation and you may be asked to present a topic, join a group discussion or work through practical problems
Group tutorial	This may be a group of up to five students and may be used in a similar context to the seminar, but allowing greater interaction with the lecturer
Individual tutorial	You should use this as an opportunity to discuss your progress, academic interests and any problems with your lecturer. The usual focus of a tutorial is an essay or project
Workshop	This is an interactive session with greater emphasis on activity than in a seminar
Project work	Project work can emphasise the responsibility and freedom you have as a learner, as you may be able to define what you learn and the method by which you learn, within defined limits. You may work to a 'learning contract' to define your aims and learning outcomes of the project
Groupwork	Groupwork allows you to pool your knowledge and skills with other students, as well as developing your interaction and negotiation skills. Very often, groupwork involves presenting a topic to the rest of the student group

Activity

Access the VARK web site at www.vark-learn.com to identify your learning style and find out how to make the best use of it.

What is the value of knowing your preferred learning style?
If you are aware of your preferred learning style, it can help you to study more effectively by using techniques to help you understand and process information. Some of the tips below may be useful.

If you are a *visual learner*, you prefer visual information and remember things best when you have seen them, so to help you process information:

- Use pictures, charts and maps when possible.
- Use planners, organisers or goal-setting charts.
- Highlight important points by underlining or using a highlighter pen.
- Use models when they are available.
- Read and recopy notes for revision.

If you are an *auditory learner*, you learn best by listening or being involved in discussion, so to help you process information:

- Talk things through as you learn them, in a tutorial group or with friends.
- Read aloud to yourself when possible.
- You may find it helpful to experiment whether you study best with music in the background or in silence.

If you are a learner who prefers *reading and writing*, then higher education should be ideal for you! You should be able to process reading text and writing notes and essays, but you may find it useful to:

- Convert graphs, charts and diagrams to words.

If you are a kinaesthetic learner, you learn best by *doing something*, so to help you process information:

- Take plenty of breaks while studying.
- Move around as you learn and revise.

Remember that these learning styles identify your *preference* for learning only. That does not mean that they are your strengths or that you should only consider a learning style for use in all situations. It is important to work on developing a range of strategies to cope with the variety of learning situations you will encounter. You may well find your learning style will differ depending on the topic you are learning about and most of us use all four styles at certain times.

Making good use of your time

Studying for a Foundation Degree means devoting time to study as well as actually working, so you may find that giving yourself enough time to devote to studies is difficult, particularly if you have family or other commitments.

Activity

There are many texts which suggest it may be helpful to list all the things you do in a day (including evenings) for the period of a week to help you see where your time is spent. You may want to try this using a table like the one shown in Table 1.2, if you are unsure where study time is going to fit into your life. Make sure you are honest!

TABLE 1.2

	Mon	Tues	Wed	Thurs	Fri	Sat	Sun
7.00	Ironing	Sleeping					
8.00	Breakfast	Breakfast					
9.00	Children to school	Study day (College)					
10.00	Shopping						
11.00	Coffee with a friend						
12.00	Lunch						
13.00	Reading time						
14.00							
15.00	Collect children						

Completing the table should show you where there is the possibility of making study time and this can then become part of your weekly routine, though of course most of us lead busy lives and sometimes we have to adapt. You also need to think about where you can study and try to find somewhere where you can work quietly with minimum disturbance.

Use any course information provided by your lecturers to help you plan your time. You will need to work out how to meet deadlines for handing work in, as well as keeping a timetable of when you are attending taught sessions and allocating time for private study.

Tips for planning your time

1 **Make plans:** Use a planner that you feel comfortable with, such as a diary, Filofax, wall planner or electronic diary to identify important commitments, such as lectures, tutorials, seminar presentations, examinations, assignment deadlines.

It may be useful to identify different activities in differing colours and if you are a visual learner, you may want to hang your planner on the wall or stuck on the 'fridge!

2 **Organise your study time:** Organise your planner on a weekly basis depending on your deadlines and schedules. Make a note of when you have lectures and work to attend and decide how you will use unscheduled slots for reading, assignment writing, library visits, etc.

3 **Organise your personal and social time:** Make sure you have a balance between work and leisure time. You cannot work if you are too tired and you cannot expect to have no time to relax, so make sure you have time to sleep, exercise, spend some 'quality time' with the family as well as time to study. Completing a table like the one shown in Table 1.2 shows you how much time you spend at work and how much at leisure!

4 **Set priorities:** You need to decide which are the most important things to work on and which can be left for a while. Clearly, if you are preparing a seminar presentation for next week, it is more important to be working on that than revising for an examination in three weeks' time!

So, to make the best use of your time:

- **Getting started:** Set yourself clear, realistic goals. Split a big task into smaller, more manageable ones. If there are study tasks you do not like, try putting them at the start of a study session. Get them finished and reward yourself by doing things you enjoy doing.
- **Keeping going:** Try to have variety when you study, so aim not to do the same thing hour after hour. Break up long study sessions with a walk to review your progress and then come back to work feeling refreshed.
- **Know when to stop:** When you have achieved the goal you set for yourself, stop and reward yourself. Take some time to do something interesting but not essential. Do not start a new task if you do not think you have time or energy to complete it.
- **Know what gets in your way:** If there are things that get in your way such as noise, poor concentration, distractions such as the family or housework, be active in overcoming them by choosing where you study and sticking to your schedule.

What should you study?

Now you have identified space and time for study, it is important to set about studying the right things. Make the most of materials given out accompanying each module or unit of study, such as course handbooks and module guides.

These will contain *learning outcomes or objectives*, which you can use to identify the depth and breadth of an area you will study. You will notice that these contain descriptive words such as 'describe', 'analyse', 'evaluate', 'list', which should indicate the amount of detail you should give to the topic. (We will cover this area again in looking at essay writing.)

As well as identifying learning outcomes or objectives, the module guide should also provide a reading list for the module. This will be a list of resources you should aim to be familiar with in order to be able to address the module content and to be prepared for the module assignment. The resources may be a list of books, journals, TV programmes/videos and web-based materials. Clearly, if a substantial list were provided you could not possibly read all the items, but you should be familiar with the set texts or the recommended texts for the module. You also need to identify which texts you wish to buy as your own copy, rather than rely on borrowing from the library what are going to be very popular books.

The set or recommended textbook(s)

The set textbook or recommended texts are important and you should know how to make the best use of them. Take time to look all through them and identify how they are made up. Many textbooks follow one of the patterns identified in Table 1.3.

Activity

Check the recommended set texts for your course and identify the different sections shown above.

Do not forget that library staff will know the usual books and journals used by your course, so always make the most of the staff by asking questions and seeking their advice on literature searches! You may find that some set texts are so popular you will only find them in the reference section or short-loan section of the library.

Where to start finding information for your course

Lecturer notes and reading lists are clearly the most important source of identifying the information you need to find in order to address the course content

TABLE 1.3   *UNDERSTANDING THE STRUCTURE OF A TEXTBOOK*

Cover	Cover	Cover
Title and subtitle	Title and subtitle	Title
Publisher and date	Publisher and date	Publisher and date
Table of contents	Table of contents	Contents
Chapters	Chapters	Chapters
Notes	Notes	Notes
Further reading	Bibliography	References
Index	Index	Appendices

Contents and index	The contents page and the index are usually positioned as above and are very useful because they help you to track down what you want from the book very quickly. Speed read both initially to identify relevant information and then once you have found it, you can focus on it to get more detail
Chapter headings	The chapter headings provide a more structured way of finding what you want and you should take time to read them carefully. These enable you to focus on your area of study and may well be important to answer your assignments. Once you have established this core, you can start to consider further reading
Further reading	The further reading page(s) of a textbook are just that – suggested titles of other textbooks, journals or web pages that can broaden your knowledge of a subject. Further reading can be read alongside the bibliography and references to identify other related texts and this can save time searching in the library
Notes	Notes usually refer to other references made in the chapter such as explanations of vocabulary. The appendix (plural appendices) will be referred to at certain points in the text and will point you to another body of information which may be a list of items, an explanation or a document

and be prepared for assignments. You will probably also carry out a web search using an appropriate search engine (this is discussed more fully in Chapter 3), but you need to take care that Internet sources are relevant and you can trust the academic credibility and author of such articles. You must, though, make use of appropriate books (and probably in the later stages of your course, journals) as web sources alone are unlikely to give your work sufficient academic 'depth'.

Once you have located a text, you need to evaluate it. Is it worth using your precious library allowance on it?

- Check the introduction and conclusion, which will tell you the purpose and scope of the book and what kind of student it is written for. Is it right for you?
- Is it written at the right academic level? Check the index, references and bibliography – if any of these are missing it may not be scholarly enough for your purpose.
- The author – is he or she a known authority on the subject? Is it written from a particular theoretical or ideological perspective? If so, you must be aware of this (check with tutors if you are unsure).
- Was this book recommended by a lecturer? If so use it – especially if he or she wrote it or edited it.
- What is the date of publication? Is there a more recent edition of the book or is there a journal article with more recent information on the topic? Remember that books contain information that may be two years old before they are even published, but journals may have information which is only six months old.

If you decide to take the book out of the library, you need to make the best use of it you can as quickly as possible. Do not forget that other students on your course may also want to read the book and it can be recalled at any time, reducing the amount of time you can keep it for.

As you read the book, keep the following points in mind, but remember that different strategies work best for different people so try different approaches until you find ones which 'work' for you:

- Set yourself a time limit, per page, per chapter, per book. Keep to the time limit by using your watch and your planner to make sure you do not slip behind your schedule.
- Reading the text for the first time means you should 'skim read' it. This means you need to train your eyes to see more. Usually when we read, we see only two or three words at a time, but with skim reading, you need to start reading from the middle of the page or in a zigzag so that you are taking in more words at once. Once you get used to this, it is easier to get a sense of what each page is about quickly. Key words will become obvious to you so that you can make a note of going back to that passage to read it in more detail later.
- If you find it difficult to skim read, perhaps because you have dyslexia, you may find 'ladder reading' helpful. This is taking the first line of each paragraph to get an understanding of the passage which should then give you a sense of the whole piece.
- Try to avoid going back over a sentence if you are speed reading. Make sure you keep to your time limit.
- Always remember *why* you are reading the book. It is easy to get bogged down in detail and forget the real reason for reading that section. If you come across unfamiliar words, make a note of them and their definitions to help you remember.
- Although it is slower, you may find it helpful to read out loud, particularly if the ideas you are reading about are unfamiliar. Reading out loud helps us to process information more quickly and as we only tend to remember a tenth of what we read, it is a more active way of absorbing information.
- You may also find it helpful to be asking questions of what you read: what are the main points of this chapter? Is the content believable? Is it of value for my assignment?

Reading skills

Reading is a vitally important activity in working towards your Foundation Degree and it needs to form a part of your weekly schedule. Try also to get into the habit of always having reading material with you so that you can dip into a book or article at any time, whether you are making a train journey, waiting at the dentist for your appointment, or sitting in the car waiting to collect the children from school!

We have already outlined the importance of using reading techniques to get the most out of library sources as quickly as possible. Five more ways you can improve your reading are as follows.

Checking your style of reading

Styles of reading can be changed to suit the situation in which we are reading:

- Scanning, for a specific focus: This is the technique we use when we are looking for a name in the telephone directory. We move our eyes quickly up and down the lists of names until we see one that looks familiar and then focus in until we find the name we want. In the same way, scan reading means we are moving our eyes quickly over the page until we find words or phrases that match what we are looking for. It may be particularly useful to scan the introduction or preface of a book, the first or last paragraphs of chapters, and the concluding chapter of the book, to see if they are going to be useful to you. Scan the abstract section of a journal article, to see if it is worth reading the whole article.
- Skimming, for getting the gist of something: This is the technique we use when going quickly through a newspaper or magazine – we tend to pick out the main points but miss out the details. It is useful to skim read a passage before deciding whether to read it in detail, or to refresh your understanding of a passage after you have read it in detail. We suggested earlier that skimming is important when choosing a book in the library or bookshop and deciding if it is the right one for you.
- Detailed reading, for extracting information accurately: This is when you read every word of the text and work to learn from the text. This technique calls for careful reading, so you may find it helpful to skim read it first, identifying if there are any words you are unsure of and may need to use a dictionary for. You can use Post-it notes to mark pages you need to concentrate on rereading. Then go back and read it in detail, making sure you understand all the points that are raised.

Become an active reader

Reading for your course is not the same as reading a novel. You need to be actively involved with the text and making notes to help your concentration and understanding. Tips to help with active reading:

- Underlining and highlighting: You can do this with your own books or photocopies but not on borrowed books! Make sure you make a photocopy first and use a highlighter pen or underline parts of the text you consider to be the most important. If you are a visual learner, you may find it helpful to use different colours for different aspects of your work – but take care you do not end up highlighting whole paragraphs as this is a waste of effort.
- Note key words: To do this you need to record main headings as you read and then add one or two key words for each section of the text. You could do this by writing in the margin of the text or keeping a notebook with you as you read.
- Questioning what you read: You need to have some idea of the questions you want the text to answer before you start reading and note these down. You can then add the answers from the text as you read. This also focuses your reading into key areas.
- Summaries: Pause after you have read a section and make a note of what you have read in your own words. You can then skim through the section again and fill in any gaps left in your notes.

Speed up your active reading

We hope you will have realised how important it is to learn from reading. You can train your mind to be active by using the SQ3R technique, which stands for *Survey, Question, Read, Recall* and *Review*.

Survey

Get together the information you need to focus on your work:

(a) Read the title to help prepare for the subject.
(b) Read the introduction or summary to see what the author thinks are the key points.
(c) Notice the bold face headings to see what the structure is.
(d) Take note of graphs, charts or tables – they are usually helpful.
(e) Notice the reading aids, italics, bold face, questions and activities in the chapter – they are usually there to help you remember and understand.

Question

Use the headings in the text as questions you think each section should answer. This means your mind will be actively engaged in trying to find answers.

Read

Read the first section looking for answers to your questions. Make up new ones if necessary.

Recall

After each section, check that you can answer your questions, preferably from memory.

Review

Once you have finished the chapter, go back and see if you can answer all the questions. If not, go back and refresh your memory.

Spot signposts for reading

As you get used to a writer's style, you should be able to recognise how the writer sets out work to give you a signpost of what is to follow in the text. A couple of examples are:

- 'Three advantages of ... ' or 'A number of methods are available ... ' should lead you to expect several points to follow.
- The first sentence of a paragraph may lead you to a sequence 'One important cause of ... ' followed by 'Another important factor ... ' and so on, until 'The final cause of ... '.

You can take advantage of this style of writing when skimming and scanning and use each point as a question in SQ3R.

Broaden your use of words and vocabulary

You will always come across new words when you are reading and it may not be that the context in which they are used will give you enough information to be able to understand them. If you do not know what they mean, how to use them and how to say them, then you will only ever be able to use words you are familiar with!

You need to be able to use technical words or jargon associated with your subject area. Write the words down, look up their meanings and find out how to pronounce them.

To do this, it is worth investing in a dictionary, preferably not a 'concise' or 'compact' one, but one which will not only show you how to spell a word but also give you:

- Alternative definitions
- Derivations (where the word comes from)
- Pronunciation (can be really useful in preparing for a seminar or presentation)
- Synonyms (words which have similar meanings, such as shut and close) and confusables (words which seem to be the same but actually are different such as affect and effect, advice and advise).

You may also find a thesaurus useful as this can help to make the language you use more varied by giving you alternative words with the same meaning. Another way of increasing your vocabulary is by reading a 'quality' newspaper at least twice a week and being sure you treat the reading as you would a piece of text, using the techniques above.

Taking notes and making use of them

In talking about reading skills, the importance of your being an active learner and using questions and notes to engage with your reading to help your concentration, your understanding and remember more of what you read, has already been identified. The same is true of notes made at lectures and seminars, which should be an active process for learning.

Activity

Take a few moments to reflect on how you currently make notes at a lecture or seminar. Think about:

o   What is achieved by making notes?
o   What uses do you have for your notes?
o   Where and how do you keep your notes after the session?

Making notes is going to be an invaluable part of your day at college or university, because they form a vital part of the information you need for your course. They create some order to your sessions and you probably label them with the session number, the lecturer's name and the date. They record your progress through lectures and texts and provide revision notes for assignments and examinations.

You may be a student who does not believe it is necessary to make notes since the lecturer invariably gives a handout for the session and all you have to do is turn up to the session and listen. However, it is rare for a handout to contain all the information imparted during a lecture and it is very difficult to concentrate on what is being said for up to an hour unless you are actively involved in learning.

Making the most of lectures

Lectures are used at college or university for two main purposes:

• to give an overview of the subject, which means you need to fill in the detail; and
• to give detailed information on a topic, which means you will need to fill in the background.

In both instances, you will note that lectures will not give you the full amount of information you need to know about the topic area or to prepare for assignments. You are expected to read around the lectures to supplement the information provided by your lecturer.

Preparing for lectures

Your module guide should identify the order in which your lectures will be delivered to you and any reading associated with each session. Doing some preparatory reading will make it easier for you to follow the lecture and also allow you to judge more easily how detailed your notes need to be.

During the lecture

Obviously the most important role in the lecture is for you to listen to what is said. However, active learning is the most effective, so note taking is also important and this means you need to be in a place where you can see and hear what is going on and away from distractions. The skill of note taking in a lecture is to summarise what has been said or written in a clear, concise form and with no facts left out, so you need to consider the best way of making notes.

Be selective

Note taking does not mean writing down everything you see or hear. Your notes need to be a summary of essential points of a text or a lecture, so you need to be selective about what you write down.
   Notes should help you to:

- Remember what was said.
- Fix information in your mind.
- Use information for assignments.
- Revise when necessary.

Find out what the lecture is about

Apart from the date and title, do not try to write anything at the start of the lecture. Listen to find out what the content is going to be and maybe write down key words and ideas which do not have to be in complete sentences. This way you have an idea of the direction the lecture will be taking and you can supplement the key words with other notes as the lecture progresses.

Find the best way of recording information

Some students always use 'linear notes', but these are best used when there is progression to the topic area, such as the example shown in the box.

Anaemia
<u>Definition</u>

Anaemia is the lack of oxygen-carrying capacity of the blood

A. Types of anaemia
B. Problems caused by anaemia
C. Implications for care for a person with anaemia

A.i) Iron deficiency anaemia
     Iron deficiency anaemia is ....

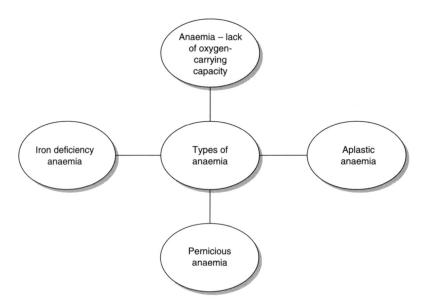

Figure 1.1   *Example of diagrammatical notes*

Some students find it more helpful to use diagrammatical notes, such as mind maps or spidergrams. These can be particularly helpful to visual learners, such as the example shown in Figure 1.1.

Use abbreviations in notes

You should get used to using common abbreviations to save yourself time as you write. Some of these are as follows:

eg	for example
nb	note well
ie	that is
cf	compare
=	equals
>	greater than
<	less than
C19	19th century
∴	therefore
∵	because
→	leads to

You may also find you use your own abbreviations to speed up writing. For example, 'pts with anaemia have ↓ Hb, → SOBOE', which translates to 'patients with anaemia have a low haemoglobin level which causes shortness of breath on exertion' (haemoglobin is the protein in blood which carries oxygen in the red blood cell). Whichever abbreviations you use, make sure you can understand your notes afterwards!

Make the most of handouts

Many lecturers give out handouts in lectures, often before they start to speak. There may be spaces left on the handout for you to fill in your own notes and supplement the lecture slides or it may be left up to you to 'customise' the notes by using highlighters or pens to pick out key points, note meanings of words in the margins or note a reference for further reading. This will help you to be an active learner so you will remember you have read them and show the key points of the session straightaway when you come back to them.

After the lecture

Whichever method of note taking you use, it is important to do something with your notes and make sure they can be used in the future. If you took notes to extend your memory, you need to be sure you can retrieve the information. It is easy to end up with large piles of notes (a piling system rather than a filing system!), which can happen if you store all your notes in the same file or use the same notebook for all modules. Key points after the lecture are to:

- Go through your notes within 24 hours of making them, while the lecture is still fresh in your mind.
- Tidy up your notes and make them legible if you need to.
- Pick out key points with highlighters or marker pens and make sure key references can be found.

- Summarise your notes if you need to, especially if you will need to revise these notes for an exam.
- Fill in your notes with examples and facts which you would not have had time to note in the lecture.
- Follow up any key points with reading and check out issues in your textbooks.
- Check out any points you do not understand with your friends or ask the lecturer before the beginning of the next session.
- Revise your notes before the following week's lecture so you can be reminded of the topic.

Writing essays

Writing essays or assignments are a very common form of assessment in higher education. The topic for an assignment is usually set as soon as a new module is launched, with an identification of the required number of words and the academic style needed.

Essay writing gives you an opportunity to:

- Explore a topic in detail by reading widely around a subject.
- Develop skills for producing an academic argument.
- Demonstrate that you can identify and use evidence to support your arguments.
- Tackle a topic in a new and original way.

Clearly, essay writing is an essential skill for all undergraduate students. Many of the problems students encounter arise from either leaving the writing of the essay until far too late in the module, or not really addressing what is required for the essay. The actual sitting down to write the essay comes quite late in the process: there is a considerable amount of preparatory work to be undertaken first.

Read the question

This seems so basic, but it is really important to appreciate how each word in an essay title makes a difference to the way it is answered. See the examples below:

Discuss the use of good interpersonal skills in a care context.

Explain the use of good interpersonal skills in a care context.

The first example expects the assignment to contain arguments for and against the use of interpersonal skills, with examples of how they can affect the relationship with a person. The second example would only expect you to state what good interpersonal skills are and account for them.

So, by misreading or misinterpreting just one word, the assignment content could be completely different and at least 50 per cent of the marks would be missed.

Some other key words (sometimes called the 'descriptors') used in essay titles are identified in Table 1.4. It is important you have a good understanding of them.

TABLE 1.4   *KEY WORDS USED IN ESSAYS*

Account for	Give an explanation of why something is the way it is
Analyse	Examine the subject in detail, breaking it down into sections to identify how and why
Argue	Make the case for something
Assess	Evaluate something, using evidence to support assessments
Comment on	Write explanatory notes, giving a view on
Compare	Consider the similarities (and sometimes differences) between two things
Contrast	Put two things in opposition to expose the similarities and differences between them
Criticise	Make judgements about the merits of theories, supported by evidence
Define	Give the exact meaning of a word, phrase or concept
Describe	Provide a full and detailed account of something
Discuss	Investigate and explore the arguments for and against something
Evaluate	Make an appraisal of the worth of something, supported by evidence
Explain	Interpret and account for something
Illustrate	Use a figure or diagram to explain or clarify, or make clear by using examples
Justify	Give reasons for decisions and conclusions
Outline	Give the general principles of a subject
Prove	Demonstrate or establish the truth or accuracy of something, using evidence
Summarise	Give a concise account of, omitting details and examples
Trace	Follow the development or history of a topic

Make sense of the question

A major part of preparing to answer an essay question is researching around the topic and reading. Therefore, it makes sense to be sure you understand what the question asks you to do.

Here is an example of a question and how it can be made sense of:

Older adults should be the responsibility of the social care system rather than the health service. Discuss.

Firstly, you could put a box around the activity words, by looking at what the question asks you to do. In this case, it is 'discuss'.

Then you could underline the key things the question asks you to discuss. In this case it is 'Older adults', 'responsibility', 'social care' and 'health service'.

It is important to look at the words which are not underlined to see if it makes a difference if they are not included. In this instance, the word 'should' makes a big difference to the meaning of the essay.

Finally, you may find it helpful to make a grid and as items from your reading uncover issues relating to the different arguments you are making, you can add them to the appropriate square:

	For	Against	Should
Social care			
Health			

Read for the essay

The previous section identified some tips for reading texts and making notes. In order to prepare for your essay, make sure you take note of the following:

- Check your guidelines. What is the word limit? What is the hand-in time? Are there any requirements for writing style, font, references, etc.?
- Select materials. Always keep the question in mind as you start to read. Make sure you use lecture notes, handouts and recommended reading.
- Move to more detailed texts. Go on to look at articles in journals, references in handouts, references in selected texts and an Internet search if required.

Make a plan of the essay

Once you are clear about the essay title and have done some background reading, you are ready to plan the essay. You probably have a number of ideas and planning should help to put these ideas into some sort of logical order before you start to write.

Your ideas may need to be sorted into two sections, *argument* and *evidence*.

The *argument* is a summary of your answer to the question. It should develop throughout the essay, with every point building on the one before. The main argument is the core of the essay and will probably only be about five or six sentences. However, each sentence will need to be explained and will need to be supported by evidence. You may also need to introduce arguments which conflict with the sentence, so that you can explain why one view is not as watertight as another.

The *evidence* is the material you use to back up your argument. This is the result of your reading and may consist of facts, material from set texts, other peoples' ideas, and so on. The evidence to support your essay and your analysis of it will form the bulk of the essay. However, always remember that it is there to support your argument and you will need to explain why you are introducing it as evidence and its role in the argument. This is known as sign-posting and can be likened to a barrister identifying why he or she is calling a particular witness to the stand to testify in a case.

The plan can be written however you like – so long as it makes sense to you and allows you to add enough detail to be realistic. Some lecturers will accept a draft of a plan to see and give advice on before you set about writing the essay properly, so it needs to be understandable to them as well. You could write your plan as a mind map – particularly helpful if you are a visual learner. Fill a whole sheet of paper with your ideas of how the essay should be structured and use different colours or highlighter pens to link points. Or it could be a series of numbered points with an item of argument and supporting evidence attached. Or you could identify each point on an index card, which could con-tain cross-references to other work or important quotations, and then arrange these in various sequences until you feel you have the order that works best. You can then number them before you start to write.

Write the essay

Finally you are ready to write the essay – or at least, the first draft of the essay. You may find yourself following the route identified in Figure 1.2 before you are happy with a final submission of your work:

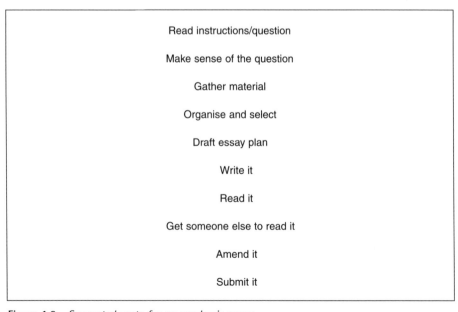

Read instructions/question

Make sense of the question

Gather material

Organise and select

Draft essay plan

Write it

Read it

Get someone else to read it

Amend it

Submit it

Figure 1.2   *Suggested route for an academic essay*

Style of writing for the essay

Academic essays usually ask for a formal style of writing which is in the third person; that is, the essay does not use 'I', 'we' or 'you'. It is generally also unacceptable to identify gender. The only exceptions to these rules may be if you are asked to write a personal diary or a piece of reflective writing.

Examples are given in the box of unacceptable and acceptable writing styles:

Unacceptable style	Preferred academic style
During this essay, I will discuss three factors which can influence health. The factors I have chosen are diet, smoking and exercise.	During this essay, three factors which can influence health are discussed. These factors are diet, smoking and exercise.
During the assessment interview, the carer should ensure she allows time for the patient to ask questions. If the patient is confused it may be necessary to ask one of his relatives to confirm details.	During the admission interview, the carer should allow time for the person to ask questions. If the person is confused it may be necessary to ask a relative to confirm details.

What should be the content of an essay?

Academic essays should be made up of three components: an introduction, a conclusion and a main body or the main content.

The introduction

The introduction has two main functions:

• It focuses the reader's attention on the central themes of the essay and should pick up some of the key words from the essay title.
• It should give the reader some understanding of the order in which you are going to develop your ideas throughout the essay.

This introduction links up with some words from the title of the essay and uses signposting to tell the reader what to expect in the essay.

You may find it preferable to write the introduction at the end, when you have already developed your arguments. To do this, though, you need to be sure you have a good plan to work from.

The conclusion

The conclusion also has two main functions:

- It pulls together and summarises details of the arguments you have been developing throughout the essay.
- It refers the reader back to the essay title, demonstrating that you have answered what you were asked to answer.

The main rules for the conclusion are:

- Do not be tempted to add new material in the conclusion.
- Do not end your assignment with a quote.
- Do not make the conclusion more than a couple of paragraphs long.

The main content

The main content is the application of the argument and the evidence referred to earlier. Remember that the academic essay is not a narrative; that is, it is not just a series of facts. Your aim is to construct an argument by showing that you can use knowledge, not just have it. This is why it may take some practice and several drafts of an essay before you feel ready to submit it.

The main areas to consider when writing the main content of the essay are:

- Relevance of the material used: Make sure you read the title of the essay carefully and make sense of it before you start to search for related reading material.

  Check your essay guidelines and look to see if the lecturer has given pointers for how you should address the essay or the amount of breadth and depth you should cover.
- Using written sources: Writing an academic essay provides written evidence of your ability to research a topic, produce arguments, organise your thoughts in a logical, coherent and critical manner and reach a suitable conclusion. You will not be able to do that unless you carry out wide and critical reading, understanding and evaluating as you read.

  Make sure you use at least the set text for the essay, but depending on the level of the work, use at least another six sources and relevant, up-to-date journal articles.

  Where possible, avoid using direct quotes in your work. Paraphrasing gives you the opportunity to use more than one author's opinion and demonstrates your ability to analyse others' work, not just to copy it.
- Making a reasoned argument: Your essay needs to be logical and fluent. Sometimes, your guidelines will advise you that you are allowed to use subheadings, but most often your work will be a continuous piece of writing. This means it must:

  (a) Make connections between points and points of view.
  (b) Link the discussion to the essay title, the introduction and the main theme of the essay.
  (c) Not be your point of view; it must be supported by relevant evidence.

This really is the importance of using signposts in the essay. If you are making up furniture from a flat pack and do not follow the written instructions in the correct order, you may end up making a wardrobe instead of a table!

Similarly, in our example essay, paragraphs will need to be written to address the issues of: what is considered to be an older adult and how this perception has changed over the last few generations; how older people have traditionally been cared for by the family and how the family structure is changing in today's society; what the medical model is and its view of the older adult; what independence for an older person means and the advantages and disadvantages to the older person of continuing to live in the community; and so on. Each topic area needs to be supported by evidence from reading, reinforced and then the next topic area moved to.

You need to read through and check how the meaning of one point relates to another. Does it: support it? Contradict it? Lead on from it? You can link one to the other by phrases such as:

(a) Consequently, it may be seen that …
(b) As a result, it can be concluded that …

which show how one thing occurs as a result of another.

(c) By contrast …

expresses a change of direction.

(d) However …

suggests an alternative viewpoint.

(e) Despite the fact that …
(f) Although it has been demonstrated that …

give the opportunity to offer additional evidence or suggest there is another way of seeing the argument.

Another helpful tip is to check the first sentence of every paragraph. Does it relate to the question? If not, is it relevant?

• Making sure the standard of presentation is good: Having put so much work into preparing your essay, why risk putting the marker in an instantly bad mood because you had not checked the presentation? It takes just a few extra minutes to read through your work, making sure that it makes sense, that the ideas flow logically, that it is interesting, that you have used a wide vocabulary and that the spelling and referencing are correct. Make sure you have used the correct size font, left margins and have an extra copy of your work.

It is worthwhile reading your work aloud to check the length of sentences, to make sure you have used a mix of present tense and any other tense and that you have not made any unintentional repetitions or puns.

Many of us use a spell-checker on the computer but incorecty speled words can distracte the reeder from the content of you're essay. It is important that you cheque you're work thoroughly fore any unecesry spelling mistakes.

Activity

The following sentence does not contain spelling errors, but clearly does not make sense! Proofread it to make sense of it:

Phil run too the hose and opened the poor. She was prized that no one was at dome. Fortunately, he new were the keys are kept, and could drove him self to hospital if necessary. He stooped in front off the mirror and raw blood ripping down his lace.

Keeping your eye on the time!

Essay writing is a time-consuming skill and one which requires practice. Make sure you allow plenty of time to go through all the stages identified and, if possible, have some sleep before you look critically at your final draft again, before you submit it.

And make sure you can rely on your computer and your printer not to let you down – a technical error like running out of ink will not usually be an acceptable reason for late submission of work.

Writing a report

Writing a report requires a very different writing style to writing an essay. You may be required to write at least one report during your Foundation Degree, possibly to write up an investigation or an aspect of work-based learning.

A report is different to an essay in three main ways, as shown in Table 1.5.

TABLE 1.5   *KEY FEATURES OF A REPORT*

In purpose	A report needs to conclude with clear recommendations about what action is suggested as a result of the findings; an essay, particularly a discussion, may conclude that further investigation is required
In structure	A report has headed and numbered sections, with an index in front, and may contain one or more appendices; most essays are a continuous piece of writing
In style	A report will always be written in the third person, avoiding 'I' or 'we'; some essays may encourage use of personal pronouns

You will probably be given a standard format for your report to follow which may be contained in the academic guidelines for your college or university. It is most important that you follow the guidelines as marks are usually awarded for the layout as well as the content of the report and the ease with which relevant information can be found. That means paying particular attention to headings, subheadings, margins and the spacing of sections.

A typical standard report structure is identified in Table 1.6.

TABLE 1.6   *STRUCTURE OF A REPORT*

Title page	This shows the report title, author's name, date, the person or organisation for whom the report has been written
Summary	The summary needs to be at the beginning of the report to be easily accessible
	It should be written as an abstract of the whole report (including the conclusion and recommendations) so cannot be written until last
Contents page	This has a particular style – see next section
Introduction	This should be brief – usually only one paragraph
	It may include:
	• Terms of reference
	• Aims and objectives
	• Methods of investigation
	• Background information
	• Definitions of any key terms
Main body of the text	This is the substance of the report and should be divided into sections to identify how the investigation was carried out and what are the findings
	Organise it logically with headings, but keep to essential information only
	Use figures, graphs, diagrams to explain points
Conclusion	Draw together the findings, avoiding the introduction of new material
Recommendations	Identify the recommendations that appear from the previous chapters and place them in a numbered list. This may be the first section to be read, so it needs to make sense independently
References	List all references used
Appendices	Include any documents or information which add to the reader's understanding of the report

The contents page of the report

The contents page should be placed after the title page and summary. It should list all sections of the report including introduction, conclusion, recommendations and appendices. Sections within the main body of the text should be given appropriate headings and identified in the contents page.

Any charts, graphs and tables need to be listed and the appendices should also be identified separately.

There are two main ways to number chapters or sections in the contents page:

- Alpha-numeric

		Page
	Summary	1
1	Introduction	2
2	First chapter heading	3
	a) Section heading	3
	i) Subheading	5
	ii) Subheading	6
⋮		⋮
12	References	50

- Decimal

		Page
	Summary	1
1	Introduction	2
2	First chapter heading	3
	2.1 Section heading	3
	2.1.1 Subheading	5
	2.1.2 Subheading	6
⋮		⋮
12	References	50

Using references and bibliographies

Citing sources and referencing them are vitally important in any academic work. This means identifying where the evidence supporting your work comes from to ensure both you and the marker of your work can find it again. Failure to reference your work may result in the academic offence of plagiarism, which is discussed later.

Citing sources

You should be provided with academic guidelines from your college or university for the precise way in which you should use references. However, in general, the following types of sources should be cited if used:

- Direct quotes.
- Paraphrases – text which has been rewritten but is still essentially drawn from someone else's work.
- Statistics.
- Studies.
- Theories and ideas.
- Interpretations of events which are not one's own.
- Facts which are not common knowledge.

You need to cite your sources in two different places: firstly, the point at which a document is referred to in the text of your work; and secondly in a list at the end of the work. The precise way in which you do this will vary between institutions and you need to find and use the specific guidelines which apply to your course.

Plagiarism

Plagiarism is the act of taking and using another person's ideas and presenting them as if they were your own. This is regarded in academic terms as stealing. In order to avoid being found guilty of plagiarism, you must be certain that the reader can distinguish your work from the work of others, so it is essential you reference your work accurately.

Plagiarism is not just about copying an assignment from another student or author. It may also refer to items such as audio-visual work, software programs, Internet articles, an electronic journal, graphics, diagrams or a person's web site without acknowledgement of the source.

Therefore, plagiarism includes:

- Submitting work as if it were your own which has been wholly or partially drawn from other sources without citation.
- Work prepared by someone other than yourself, purchased or otherwise.
- Identical or highly similar work submitted by different students; and work originally prepared for submission elsewhere. This means that if you use the same work for an assignment elsewhere on the course, you are plagiarising your own work!

Activity

In each of the examples below, identify:

(a) Whether the students are guilty of plagiarism or if there is another reason for their actions.

(b) Why you made your decision and what the student(s) should have done.

Identifying examples of plagiarism

1   Susie submits her first essay for marking. It uses some large chunks of text from a textbook that the lecturer recommended. There are sections that are copied out word for word without the use of quotation marks. There are no references to the text in the essay but it is listed in the references at the end of the work.

2   John, Jason, Jane and Jamilla have worked together on a project and they have been asked to submit an individual account of the work as an assignment. Jane, Jamilla and John submit work with whole sections which are almost identical.

3   Mustaffa, a final-year student, hands in his dissertation which refers to a large number of sources. He has included many in-text references and quotes. There are several sections which come from an Internet site that have not been referenced.

You may have considered the following:

Example 1: Susie has obviously tried to follow the assignment guidelines and has used the text recommended by the lecturer. However, she clearly misunderstands how to cite references, since she has used the material from the book in the text but not used quotation marks or written the name of the author in the text. It is poor academic practice to use lengthy quotations, but if the original author's words are used word for word, they must be acknowledged by a reference.

You may decide that Susie has demonstrated poor academic skills since this is the beginning of her course. She needs to check her academic guidelines on referencing and try to avoid using long quotations in essays.

Example 2: Jane, Jamilla and John have not followed the project guidelines, because they were asked to submit individual pieces of work. They have plagiarised because they have submitted identical copies of work.

You may decide that they need more guidance on how to work in a group but to keep their own notes and avoid working on drafting the essay together, before the work is resubmitted.

Example 3: Mustaffa is a final-year student submitting a dissertation and should therefore be very familiar with academic rules for the submission of work. He has referenced correctly in the text but has made omissions in citing his Internet sources.

At such a stage in the course, Mustaffa has no excuse for not referencing correctly. He will be penalised and needs to consult his referencing guidelines before resubmission.

SUMMARY

- Studying for a Foundation Degree means you need to organise yourself sufficiently well to manage your work time and your study time. You will find it helpful to follow some tips to improve your learning skills and learn *how* to learn. It is never too late to improve your study skills!

- Learning how to learn includes managing time, developing effective reading and writing skills, identifying how to prepare and write essays and reports, and demonstrating how to cite sources to ensure your work is referenced and avoids plagiarism.

- It is worthwhile taking time to explore your resources for study in terms of time, space and what your course requirements are.

- It is helpful to identify your preferred learning style and try to make the most of your study time by using the resources that suit you best.

- Always read information supplied by your university or college, to ensure you follow guidelines when preparing and presenting written work for assessment.

Further reading

Burns, T. and Sinfield, S. (2003) *Essential Study Skills: The Complete Guide to Success at University*. London: Sage. An excellent and easily readable book brimming with ideas and activities on how to approach studying.

Cottrell, S. (2003) *Skills for Success*. Basingstoke: Palgrave Macmillan. This book was written primarily to assist students to meet personal development planning requirements. It is full of advice for students in higher education who want to capitalise on their learning experiences and start to prepare for the world of work.

Arksey, H. and Harris, D. (2007) *How to Succeed in your Social Science Degree. London: Sage.* A thoughtful and insightful book with a focus on the actual experience of being a student.

Many universities and colleges produce their own study skills guidance and advice for students and these are often available to use whether or not you are enrolled on a course with the university. Some noteworthy sites worth visiting are: Southampton University, The Open University, The University of Plymouth with Bournemouth University which has a specific homepage for Foundation Degree students. There are downloadable documents and links to other sites for study skills.

2 WORK-BASED LEARNING/REFLECTIVE PRACTICE

Graham Brotherton and Steven Parker

SUMMARY CHAPTER CONTENTS

- Work-based learning and placement
- Entering the workplace
- Reflecting on practice
- Developing a framework of reflection
- Reflection and empowering practice: praxis and Paulo Friere

---

Learning objectives

By the end of this chapter, you should be able to:

■ Understand the concept of work-based learning and its role within Foundation Degrees and other courses in health and social care.

■ Make use of mentoring or supervision and other support within the workplace.

■ Develop a framework to reflect on your practice in work-based learning.

■ Recognise the importance of praxis and work-based learning as the practical application of values to develop empowering approaches to practice.

Introduction

Foundation Degrees are intended to provide students with the knowledge, understanding and skills that employers need. The work-based learning element or placement of your foundation degree enables you to demonstrate the knowledge and skills that will increase your employability after you graduate from your course.

Skills for Care has published National Occupational Standards in Health and Social Care, and it is these standards which specify the vocational competencies that workers are expected to demonstrate. The standards are regarded as a measure of quality and are seen as an indicator of the skill level and competency of the workforce.

The National Occupational Standards relevant for a Foundation Degree for Health and Social Care are at Level 4. You can view these at the *Skills for Care* web site.

The work-based learning on your foundation degree will provide you with an opportunity to demonstrate your practice skills. You can use the knowledge provided in the various chapters of this book to underpin and inform your practice and enable you to develop the skills you need.

This chapter explores what is meant by work-based learning and provides you with a framework to reflect upon your practice and get the most from your practice experience. To learn form work-based learning you need to be able to learn from the experience by applying your knowledge to your practice and develop your skills through a process of reflection.

Work-based learning and placement

What is work-based learning?

On one level the answer to this question is obvious: work-based learning is any form of learning which either takes place within or relates directly to your experience of the workplace. One of the distinguishing characteristics of Foundation Degrees is that they emphasise the role of work-based learning as do many other health and social care courses, so getting to grips with the practicalities of work-based learning is an important element of your course.

Your work-based learning experience or placement is likely to be an assessed component of your Foundation Degree. You may be asked to keep a learning journal to record and note how you felt about your workplace activities. This will become the basis of your reflective learning, as you will be asked to reflect upon your practice. Other assignments from other modules may require you to relate particular knowledge to your practice experience. And later, perhaps in your second year, you may be set a particular research topic related to your workplace.

In order to make the most of workplace learning you should have a placement in a work setting that you are passionate about. What area of health and social care are you concerned about? Where do you want to make that difference? To make sure you get the placement that is right for you, it is of paramount importance that you discuss placement opportunities with your course tutors. It is also important to discuss your placement with the placement supervisor to make sure that your potential placement will provide you with the practice experiences you need to demonstrate the skills you wish to develop and the knowledge you have gained from your course and make a meaningful difference to a person's life.

While on placement it is important to make the most of your practice opportunities. Use the experience to take responsibility appropriate to your role as a student on placement and take a proactive approach to seeking support from placement supervisors and college tutors so that your placement meets your learning needs.

Making the most of your mentor or practice supervisor

Activity

If you have experience of mentoring or supervision try to think about good or bad experiences – what made it 'work' or not 'work'?

   Can you use this to improve your experience of mentoring now?

While the precise arrangements will vary from programme to programme, access to some form of mentor or supervisor will be very helpful for you to get the most out of work-based learning. Mentoring can take a variety of forms from the provision of a named experienced member of staff within an organisation with a formally designated role to informal support form experienced colleagues. Though a formal mentor may be the best solution in most situations, this will not always be possible. You are strongly advised to try to make some form of mentoring or practice supervision arrangement where possible.

In most cases the college or university will also provide you with a tutor to support your work-based learning. The precise allocation of roles between mentor or supervisor will again vary between organisations but should include most of the following:

- Providing you with objective but supportive feedback on practice.
- Support and guidance as to your role in the workplace and how this evolves.
- The opportunity to discuss and develop your reflective practice skills.
- Advice on acceptable standards of both practice and, where relevant, college/university assessments.

- The opportunity to 'sound out' ideas in a non-judgemental way.
- Advice on finding relevant information inside and outside the workplace.
- An advocate who will ensure your interests and concerns are appropriately addressed.
- A positive but questioning and challenging approach to practice and professional development.

In order to facilitate this there are a number of practical things which both you and your mentor or supervisor can do to ensure that the role is effective. From a student's point of view this will include:

- Being prepared for mentoring and supervision meetings with a list of key issues you want to discuss.
- Ensuring that your mentor or supervisor is kept fully up to date about your progress and any ongoing concerns.
- Discussing your progress in an open and constructive way.
- Being prepared to accept and reflect upon constructive criticism.
- Sharing your reflective accounts and other aspects of your college/university work.

In return you should be able to expect from your placement supervisor and mentor that they:

- Make appropriate time available to you.
- Provide you with thoughtful and constructive feedback.
- Read any written material that you wish them to (though it is important that you consider how much you can realistically expect them to find time to scrutinise).
- Address any concerns that you may have in a non-judgemental way.

A constructive relationship between a mentor, supervisor and a student requires effort on both sides, a willingness to work through the inevitable difficulties which will occur and the requirement on both sides to accept that things will not always run smoothly.

There are some excellent resources to support practice or work-based learning from both the student and mentor perspectives on the 'Making Practice-Based Learning Work' web site which can be found at http://www.practicebasedlearning.org/home. htm.

You may wish to review some of the materials with your mentor; though they do have a health focus, the materials can easily be used in social care contexts.

Learner contracts/agreements

One way in which some people seek to make the process work is through the use of contracts or agreements which attempt to set out how the arrangements will be organised in terms of frequency of contact, the way supervision will be organised, how confidentiality will be managed and the practice opportunities provided to you. It can be particularly useful if the college or university is included as this provides a framework for negotiation and clarification about the specific roles of the student (and how this might overlap with your role as 'worker' where this is relevant), mentor and work-based learning support tutor. It is likely that your college or university will provide you with a hand-book that covers most of these issues.

Using the workplace as a basis for assignments

One of the challenges of work-based learning is 'capturing' the learning that does take place in order to support your college or university assignments. You can obviously utilise your learning journal, diary or any other records you keep, but these are not always easy to 'translate' into the specific requirements of academic writing. In addition there are complications about respecting con-fidentiality and how far you can use specific examples to support wider ideas about theory, policy or practice. The following guidelines may help you in doing this:

- Ensure that you respect confidentiality. While examples from the workplace are very helpful, they need to be presented in ways which do not allow any individual to be identified. It is likely that your institution will have guidance on how to present placement or workplace-related material – check with your tutor.
- Make sure that you get the balance right in terms of the level of detail for any exam-ples you use; too little detail and it is impossible for the person who will read your assignment to get a full understanding of the situation. Remember that they were not there at the time of any incident and need sufficient information to be able to evalu-ate your example and any conclusions you draw from it. On the other hand, make sure you do not go into excessive detail: this uses up valuable words where there is a word limit on a piece of work and will make your work too descriptive.
- Always think about why you are using the example and what ideas, concepts, etc., you are trying to relate it to. Take a little time to organise your example in relation to this: what are the aspects of the example that are relevant in terms of the ideas or con-cepts you are trying to explore? How can you make these links in a clear and appro-priate manner?

Using work-based learning to improve practice

As a student you are in many senses in a useful position to act as a conduit between your workplace/placement and the wider professional community. As well as using the experience you gain in the workplace for your own personal and professional development, you have the opportunity to use the knowledge and skills that you are gaining through study as a way to improve practice within the workplace, e.g. by applying an action research approach (see Chapter 3) to problems within the setting or by researching current notions of good practice with your user group in the literature. This can of course be difficult in some cases in terms of maintaining effective relationships either as a student in placement or as a worker who spends time outside the setting, but with careful and diplomatic negotiation it can be perceived as beneficial for all concerned.

Entering the workplace

While on placement you will be entering the workplace as a student and so the workplace will consist of a number of interrelated areas all of which can be important for your learning. The workplace will have its own organisational culture, with its own set of values, philosophy, ethos and policies. The organisation is influenced by a range of stakeholders including work colleagues that you may meet for the first time and later work with and the people who use the service. The physical environment of health and social care you enter may be specifically designed to provide a service or it may be in someone's personal living space in their own home or within a residential service.

The workplace environment is made up of a series of spaces some of which are public and others private. Some spaces and places may be for living, others for working and others for visiting. Some spaces may be all three. You may be working with individuals or with groups. You may find yourself in formal or informal situations. These different situations will have different rules and protocols and the different places may have different atmospheres. The time, space and place for social care is multifaceted and complex and as Pearce and Reynolds (2003) remind us, this ambiguity of social care adds to its complexity.

Activity

Spend some time thinking and reflecting upon your work-based experience or placement.

Make some notes.

Decribe your workplace:

o   What kind of service do you provide, e.g. residential or day service?
o   Who uses the service?
o   Who works there?

How diverse are your staff and service users in terms of:

o   Age
o   Experience
o   Gender
o   Ethnicity
o   Qualifications?

Identify the working environment in terms of:

o   Public space
o   Private space

and

o   Formal duties
o   Informal duties.

What happened in these areas?
Who is in these areas?
Are there staff-only areas?
Do people who use the service have any private space?
How do people's roles change between spaces?
The different places and roles that people have within them at different times demonstrate the complexity of space within the health and social care workplace.

Learning in the workplace

There are a number of ways in which we learn in the workplace. To give some examples, we learn by observing, we learn by doing, we learn through conversations with colleagues, we learn through supervision. In order to maximise workplace learning we need to find ways of collecting, reflecting upon and analysing our experiences.

Activity

Try to list five things that you have learned in the last six months which relate to work.
How did you learn them?
Who from?
What impact have they had on the way in which you approach your work?

Academic versus work-based learning

One of the problems with work-based learning is how to make effective links between the academic content of your course and your vocational experiences. The ability to link 'theory' with 'practice' is an essential skill that you need to develop.

'Academic' learning is traditionally conceived of as relating to theory, the research and evidence base underpinning ideas and concepts, the policy which may come from government and the ideas of values and moral principles, all of which are covered in this book. Vocational learning is thought of as relating to practice and the development of your practice skills. One of the key elements of Foundation Degrees is the way in which they seek to link the academic and the vocational, an approach shared with most 'professional' training in health, social care and related areas. Academic learning is often caricatured as learning by thinking and vocational learning as learning by doing. The ability to reflect upon your practice by making explicit links between your academic learning and vocational experience becomes an essential method of learning. Reflection attempts to reconcile the academic and vocational and has an emphasis on evaluating practice through theory and knowledge and then using this to refine practice.

A further element within this is that it makes explicit the concept of judgement. Decisions in health and social care are rarely clear cut: most rely on an ability to interpret information which is in itself complex and may be contested (i.e. different people may have different interpretations of what the 'facts' of a situation are and how they could or should be interpreted; this is discussed further in the context of needs assessment in Chapter 9). Judgements are therefore themselves difficult and contestable and require the ability to reflect upon situations in structured and systematic ways. The framework for reflection provided in this chapter provides a structured approach for your reflection on your work-based learning and enables you to develop the skills to be a reflective practitioner.

Reflecting on practice

The essential tool for learning in the workplace is the skill of reflecting on practice. Thinking about events with a model that provides us with different perspectives enables us to see things differently. As a character in *Dombey and Son* advises:

> how will many things that are familiar, and quite matter of course to us now, look when we come to see them from that new and distant point of view which we must all take up, one day or another? (Dickens, 1896: 398)

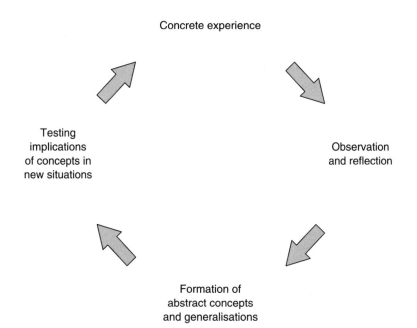

Figure 2.1   *Kolb's learning cycle (Kolb, 1984, cited in Eby, 2000a)*

The process of thinking over and reflecting on what you have done is an important part of professional development. Eby (2000a) defines reflection as enabling practitioners 'to make sense of their lived experiences through examining such experiences in context'. Reflecting on our practice is part of our 'personal commitment' to seek out answers to the questions that are raised by our practice.

Practice is an important learning experience and this experiential learning is an important aspect of a health and social care practitioner. As an individual practitioner you are an active learner and your everyday practice experience forms part of that learning.

Kolb's basic concept from his learning cycle (Figure 2.1) is that we constantly learn from our experience. We have an experience and we look back upon it. We reflect on that experience from a range of different perspectives, examining what went on in the experience.

By the process of reflection we develop a better understanding and link our actions to theoretical ideas. We may even develop our own theoretical ideas of how we need to improve our practice. From our new ideas and generalisations we then move on to new ways of working in which we test out our ideas.

Our new ideas are implemented in our practice, which in turn gives us a new experience. The process of learning becomes cyclical and we continue to learn through our experiences.

So we continually test our ideas in practice and change them in light of new experiences.

Reflection is about thinking about our actions. Initially it is our conversation with ourselves. So how do you think?

How do you think?

Let us take some time out to reflect on how we think.

Take five minutes or so to think about something that has happened today – it could be a conversation with someone at work or college or a piece of some work you where involved in.

Did you talk to yourself?

- Silently in your head
- Or out loud?

What language are you using?

- Where does your language come from?
- What perceptions and meanings are in the language you use?
- How does emotion enter into your conversation with yourself?
- Who owns the language you are using?

What form does your conversation with yourself take?

- Are you asking yourself questions?
- Are you answering and replying to yourself?
- Or are you describing the day's events in sequential order in words?

Do you think in pictures?

- Do you visualise any of the events?

Do you think in feeling?

- What emotions did you experience?
- Are you reliving the emotions?
- Are you aware of the feelings and emotions you experienced at the time?

(Continued)

Where do you think?

- Where do you think about the activities of the day?
- Where do you do your daydreaming?

Do you have time and space to reflect on the activities of the day?

Thinking becomes our tool of reflection.

Schön (1983) suggested that as practitioners we may implicitly know what we are doing. This knowing in action is made up of our abilities as practitioners to make judgements and decisions almost spontaneously. Sometimes we are unaware of how we know how to do something; we may have known at one time but cannot remember the reasoning behind our actions or we may have not have known in the first place! Whatever the reason we do things simply because we do.

This is not to say that we do not think about what we are doing. We think about our actions as we do them; this reflection in action is constant and ongoing, or we may think back over our actions, by reflecting on our action.

To improve our practice Schön says we need to reflect on our action by looking back over our practice. By reflecting on our practice we can evaluate and learn from what we have done. By reflecting on action we can acknowledge that we have reflected in action as well. We can analyse our practice, as well as our thought processes, in order to improve our practice in the future.

To reflect successfully on our practice we need to think about it in a structured way in order to evaluate, learn and improve. We also need to use this reflective process to develop as critical practitioners.

A number of different modes of reflection exist to help practitioners reflect upon their practice, which are all essentially methods for looking back on our practice. By looking at a few influential models of reflection you will be able to see which ones may be useful for you own reflection and we will be able to suggest some essential components in the process of reflecting on your practice. They all provide methods of evaluation and a way to improve or change your practice.

Jasper (2003, cited in Adams et al., 2005) sees reflection as being a three-phase sequence of 'experience–reflection–action':

- Examining and revisiting the experience by thinking about it. This involves concentrating and examining the event in the here and now or by looking back on the experience.
- Reflecting on the experience, by exploring feelings, and examining these to develop an awareness of their implications, their importance and how they effect the outcomes of our practice.
- Deciding on the action we take during the event or in the future when we encounter similar experiences.

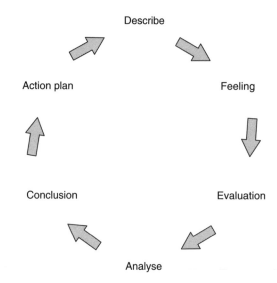

Figure 2.2   *The Gibbs reflective cycle*

Jasper's model corresponds to Schön's ideas of refection in and on action. Most models are concerned with the process of reflecting on action. The Gibbs reflective cycle (cited in Quinn, 1988) in Figure 2.2 is seen as a popular and effective framework for reflecting on your practice. It provides useful headings to write about your experience if you are keeping a reflective journal.

The first part of the cycle is to *describe* the experience. You need to describe the events. In what order did things happen? Who did what and what was said?

The *feelings* that you experienced are important. What emotions did you experience? Were you happy or pleased? Angry or upset? What made you feel this way?

To *evaluate* the experience, the Gibbs model suggests you look at the experience in terms of what was good or bad about it. What was successful and what was not?

In *analysing* the experience you need to try and make sense of what happened. Why did things happen the way they did? Were the events predictable? Were you using a particular theoretical idea to guide your actions?

By coming to a *conclusion* you need to be able to formulate ideas about their courses of action. What else could you have done in this situation? Would they have made any difference to the outcome? Can you run an alternative course of events in your reflection?

As a result of reflecting on your practice you need to have an *action plan*. If a similar situation arose again what would you do differently?

The Gibbs cycle of reflection is a useful starting place, but it seems limited in its scope for analysing your practice in depth and it does not explore the nature of thinking about complex processes and events that are informed by a rich layer of thoughts, feelings, ideas and contradictory ideas.

Boud et al. (1985) have developed a model of reflection, which attempts to deal with some of these complex and abstract ideas. The model has two main components, the experience itself and the refection on the experience. The experience includes what you thought, felt, did and the conclusions you came to about the event. This could be at the time and/or immediately after the event. The processing phase is after the event and it is here that conscious reflection takes place in three stages in which you:

- Return to the experience.
- Attend to feelings.
- Re-evaluate the experience.

Return to the experience is the retelling of the event or experience. It is important to describe the events without judgement, in chronological order. This describing of the events is so that the experience can be examined in terms of what actually happened. This seemingly detached mode of describing a situation does not mean that feelings are not acknowledged, because it is only by acknowledging both positive and negative emotions that can you move on to the next stage.

Attend to feelings is concerned with concentrating on the positive feelings associated with the event. In this model it is important to remove negative feelings as they may get in the way of reflecting on and analysing the experience in a rational way. It is not about ignoring the negative feelings and emotions, but about dealing with them so that they do not get in the way of reflecting on your practice and having creative ideas of how to develop your practice. Concentrating on the positive is also about providing the drive to persist in what may be a challenging experience.

Re-evaluate the experience in this model can only truly happen if the preceding two stages have been worked through. To re-evaluate the experience there are a further four substages to work through:

- **Association** is about making links between the ideas and feelings of the experience with your existing knowledge and values. From making these connections the idea is that you should be able to make sense of the experience and develop an understanding of the event. It is also about challenging your previous knowledge and so developing your own knowledge about a situation.
- **Integration** is concerned with making further sense of the associations you have made. After making a series of links between feelings, knowledge, attitudes and values, the idea is to sift through all this information and begin to make further sense

of it all. What connections can you make between the ideas you have generated about a particular event? What truth or insight can you come up with? What new ideas can you formulate?

- **Validation** becomes the stage where you test out your new idea. You can rehearse an event or test out a new strategy for an intervention. You do not need to test out your new idea or model in practice – you could replay and visualise the events to yourself or talk them through with someone. You need to check your new idea for any inconsistencies or contradictions. But even if your idea does not fit in with accepted practice, it does not mean that you are wrong – you could be breaking new ground.
- **Appropriation** is when the new knowledge gained from our reflections becomes your own. This may involve a fundamental change in how you work or what you believe in.

The model ends with **outcomes and action**, a new way of practice and new knowledge.

This process of re-evaluating the experience may seem quite separate from everyday practice and experience, but the value of Boud et al.'s model is that it highlights the complex and abstract nature that thinking about your practice can create. To help the process it is useful to discuss each stage in a learning set, in a tutorial, or with your practice supervisor. Another person can help with exploring the situation and making links across a range of issues.

As an alternative to this abstract model the Johns model of structured reflection (cited in Quinn, 1988) offers a series of questions and cues that you can ask yourself to guide your reflections. The questions can be used in a learning set to challenge each other so that you and your fellow learners can help each other to develop your reflective skills. The questions can also be the basis of a learning journal.

The Johns model of structured reflection

Description:

- Phenomenon – Write or give a description of the experience.
- Causal – What essential factors contributed to this experience?
- Context – What are the background factors to this experience?
- Clarifying – What are the key processes for reflection in this experience?

Reflection:

- What was I trying to achieve?
- Why did I act as I did?
- What are the consequences of my actions for:

    (a) The person and their family or carers
    (b) Myself
    (c) People I work with?

o   How did I feel about this experience when it was happening?
o   How did the person who uses the services feel about it?
o   How do I know how they felt about it?

Influencing factors:

- What internal factors influenced my decision making and actions?
- What external factors influenced my decision making and actions?
- What sources of knowledge did influence or should have influenced my decision making and actions?

Alternative strategies:

- Could I have dealt better with the situation?
- What other choices did I have?
- What would be the consequences of these other choices?

Learning:

- How can I make sense of this experience in light of past experience and future practice?
- How do I now feel about this experience?

    Have I taken effective action to support myself and others as a result of this experience? How has this experience changed my way of knowing:

- Empirics
- Aesthetics
- Ethics
- Personal?

The Johns model offers more structure than the other models outlined here and Quinn points out that such a framework could be regarded as being imposed upon practitioners. It is important to view the different models as guides to frame your reflection; the model is external to the worker and you may wish to develop your own.

Action research as a model of reflection

The notion of reflective practice is linked to the idea of action research, which is developed more fully in Chapter 3. However, it is important to note in this context that action research can be thought of as a form of formalised reflective practice with an emphasis on investigating and acting to improve elements of practice. In this sense developing an action research approach can be an important element of work-based learning and a way of linking the academic and vocational elements of your course.

Critical incident analysis

One way of developing reflective practice in a systematic way is through the use of critical incident analysis. This involves using the approach outlined above in a particularly structured way by identifying an incident of particular significance (usually something that has gone very well or very badly) and thinking the incident through in a very systematic way. This involves considering (in addition to the things outlined above):

- What context the incident or event took place in.
- How you were feeling before and after the event.
- What you were thinking at the time.
- How other people involved perceived the event or incident (in so far as it is possible to ask them).
- What the consequences were for you or the other people involved (in order to do this you need to discuss the incident with the other people who were involved).

In many cases it is useful to write this up in the form of a report and discuss it formally with a colleague (perhaps your mentor).

Activity

Try to think of a 'critical incident' within your own experience and analyse it using the model outlined above. It may be useful to record this and discuss it with you tutor or mentor.

Developing a framework of reflection

These different models of reflection and a range of others have some common elements that can be extracted and combined to develop a workable model for reflecting on your practice while undertaking your Foundation Degree. This book contains a range of information and ideas about theoretical knowledge and practice, policies and procedures, values and ethics, and the possible future for health and social care. These can be utilised to aid and develop your reflection on practice. Using the above ideas we have put together a framework that can be used with the accepted models of reflection to help guide your reflective processes.

Common to all the models of reflection is the need to describe and replay the experience, so the first thing in our guide to reflection is to:

- **Describe the experience:** Describing the situation or piece of practice is an important element in developing your reflective skills. Replay the events in a conversation with yourself or within a learning set or a tutorial group designed to aid your reflective skills. Taking on board some of the messages from the models above on how to describe the events as they happened. Recount the order of events, tell your story and write it down as soon as you can.

  In your descriptions pay attention to the minutiae of interactions, the perceived causes of behaviour, the antecedents, the behaviour and the consequences.

  It is impossible to separate out your feelings and emotions, as they are an important part of the story, so acknowledge them. You can explore the reasons why later.

  The need to attend to feelings is also part of many of the reflection models. This seems important, as identifying why you felt the way you did enables you to locate any conflicts in values, attitudes and beliefs. It may also enable you to identify areas of practice that worked well as well as pieces of work that did not go as planned. So the second part of this guide is to:

- **Acknowledge and explore your emotional responses:** How do you feel about your practice? It is important to explore how you feel about your work and what you hoped to achieve by your practice and work with people who use services. Taking elements from the Johns model, you can explore why you feel the way you do in terms of your achievements. Do you feel as if you have accomplished something or do you feel frustrated in your efforts?

  It is important to explore not only your feelings but also how other people feel and view your practice – the people who use the service you provide, fellow workers, managers, and even the organisation itself. Can you identify any conflicts between these different levels of your work?

  All the models have an element of analysis and evaluation. The Gibbs model asks you to look at your practice in terms of what was good and how you can make sense of what happened. The Boud et al. model offers us some abstract thought process to make connections and the Johns model gives us a structured set of questions. To aid your analysis and evaluation we suggest you explore your practice in the following terms:

- **Values:** It is important to be aware of your personal and professional values. Identify the values and moral principles that inform your interventions in people's lives. What are the ethical and moral dilemmas that you are encountering in your practice? Are you able to work in an empowering way and as a morally active practitioner? What is your position of power? Does this have a bearing on how you are feeling about your practice and interventions with people?

- **Theory, knowledge and practice:** It is important to identify and recognise the theories and concepts that underpin your practice. What theoretical knowledge informs your practice? Do you have a couple of favourites or is your practice heory-less?

Some of the theoretical ideas that you may be using could be suspect and open to criticism. How do you know that the knowledge you have is adequate for your practice and why are you using the theory that you do?

It is important to be able to link and use theory in your practice, but equally so it is important to be critical and not simply take theoretical ideas for granted. It is very unlikely that grand theoretical ideas can explain or inform all you actions.

*   **The policy and legal context:** Social care agencies and health authorities are bound by national and local policy, legislation and procedures. It is important to acknowledge the policies that guide your practice and the legal context in which they exist. Are you performing statutory duties and what are the legal limitations of your actions?
*   **The evidence:** An important part of reflecting on your interventions in people's lives is to be aware of the research evidence that can inform your practice. How do you know that your interventions in other people's lives will make any positive difference to their lived experience? An awareness of sound research evidence and its relevance to your practice is of paramount importance in your reflective processes, but equally so it is important to be critical of research. Ask yourself 'where is the evidence?' Is the research evidence any good? You need to question the research that is reported to underpin your practice.
*   **Where you fit in:** You need to acknowledge your role in your practice. You may have already done so by exploring your emotional responses or your personal moral principles. You could take this further to examine how you have interpreted any of these points for reflection or the meanings that you have created from reflecting on them. You are an important player when intervening in people's lives, so how have you changed someone's life course? You also need to consider how you would do things differently.

The models all have as a final outcome an aim of learning from and improving your practice. From reflecting on your practice you should be able to identify what you need for your own personal and professional development. Set yourself some objectives to develop your knowledge to inform your practice. It is in this way that you can develop as a reflective and critical practitioner.

Becoming a reflective and critical practitioner

It is not enough simply to think about your practice. As you progress through your career in health and social care it is important to develop your skills of reflective practice. This is a process of turning thoughtful practice into a learning experience. It is important to develop your skills further to become a critical practitioner and developing your reflective practice is an essential stage to work through. Your aim should be to develop an open-minded and reflective approach to your practice that considers 'different perspectives, experiences and assumptions' (Brechin, 2000; Eby, 2000a). It also becomes important to acknowledge and reflect on your personal involvement as you engage and intervene in people's lives and the relationship you have with people you provide services to.

Reflection and empowering practice: praxis and Paulo Friere

Underpinning your reflective practice should be an awareness of the values and moral principles that underpin your practice. These are explored in Chapter 5. Within this process of reflection you should be able to reflect upon your practice as its being empowering practice.

Among the most influential educational thinkers of the twentieth century, Paulo Friere emphasised the importance of dialogue in education and was very critical of many traditional approaches which he saw as a one-way process of imparting knowledge from expert teachers to passive recipients. In addition Friere saw education as explicitly concerned with change and with trying to improve the circumstances of those who are disadvantaged. It therefore needs to be underpinned by a particular and explicit commitment to values and action, known as praxis. This links explicitly with the notion of the morally active practitioner as discussed in Chapter 5.

In this model, since education should be about empowerment, there needs to be explicit reflection as to whether or not any approach or intervention is underpinned by the values which support good practice in health and social care. It can also be argued that praxis suggests that we should go a stage further and actively reflect on whether we can change our practice in ways that are commensurate with further reducing power differentials and disadvantage.

This model of praxis as informed committed practice is an important element in using workplace experience as a basis for learning. The process of linking experience to theory as a way of improving practice has a long and honourable tradition, not just in health and social care but also in related areas such as education. A key example of 'praxis' in action could be in relation to the debate around empowerment. The theoretical/moral issues about empowerment are discussed in Chapter 5.

As social care workers we are responding to the needs of people who require our services (see Chapter 9). This is undertaken under the umbrella of empowering people who use our services. Yet how far do organisations and practitioners empower people within a framework of tackling disabling barriers?

A model of empowerment based upon the social model of disability (see Chapters 5 and 9) is concerned with the breaking down of disabling barriers and the promotion of people's rights. Service users are seen as experts of their own situation and people are regarded as equal and in control of the services that are delivered. The structures and procedures of organisations need to be responsive to this. In undertaking work-based learning we need to be able to develop approaches which facilitate the empowerment of services users.

In taking account of the social model of disability practitioners need to be aware of disability issues and of the factors that create institutional discrimination. This means being aware of the attitudes and behaviour of others and ourselves and the wider structural reasons for the exclusion and marginalisation of disabled people. The disability rights movement is a social movement which campaigns for the rights of people and it is this political action that can break down the underlying reasons of disabling barriers.

But as practitioners it is important to be aware of how practice may reinforce disabling barriers. It is important to use our professional power in a way that promotes people's rights and does not reflect the disabling barriers that people face. The social model of disability is inclusive and relates to all people who face disabling barriers (Goodley, 2004).

Empowering practice

From your practice or placement you may have been involved with what is regarded as empowering practice.

This exercise enables you to explore your practice within a framework of values and empowerment, so you need to be familiar with the content of Chapter 5. You will also need to refer to the policies of the organisation and how they promote service user rights and equality.

Find and explore your organisation's mission statement and policies regarding the services it provides. You may need to access these through your agency's internal web site and electronic resources.

Evaluate the organisation's policy by referring to the social model of disability, the promotion of rights and implications of human rights legislation, the development of advocacy services and normalisation.

You could ask yourself:

o   Does the policy promote service user control of services?
o   What is the attitude expressed by the policies towards the people who receive services?
o   Are the policies that you have found accessible to people who use the services provided by the organisation?
o   Are service users regarded as passive recipients of a service or are they fully involved in organisational policy and practice as equal human beings?
o   What model of empowerment do you think is promoted by the organisation?

- o   Does the organisation truly empower service users?
- o   How does your practice fit in with organisational policy?
- o   Can you be a morally active practitioner?

It becomes important to reflect on your role as a social and health care practitioner, by looking at the wider social context of the work you are doing, the moral and ethical base of your work and your guiding moral and ethical principles. It is important to ask yourself if your practice is empowering practice.

Being morally active

Husband (1995) points out that as practitioners we need to take moral responsibility for our practice and we need to be morally active practitioners. To be morally active means that we should act on the basis of our internal values and as an autonomous moral agent. To do this successfully requires practitioners to be able to reflect upon their values and moral principles and what they believe in when working with service users. It becomes important to understand and recognise the values and moral principles that underpin our practice and this is explored further in Chapter 5.

SUMMARY

This chapter has explored how work-based learning is an essential part of your learning on your Foundation Degree and we have emphasised the practical arrangements you need to consider to ensure your practice placement provides you with the practice opportunities you need so that it is a successful learning experience.

We have covered various approaches to reflection on practice and you should be able to use the framework presented here to develop a structured approach to reflection which will enable you to make the most of work-based learning for yourself and to the placement itself.

By using the reflective models we have outlined and the framework for reflection you should be able not only to develop your knowledge and skills but also to develop your ability to engage with your practice. It is important to take into account the notions of praxis and being morally active for your continual personal and professional development.

By reflecting on your role within the workplace you should be able to develop an empowering approach to your practice and make a meaningful and positive difference to people's lives.

There is a very limited literature available on work-based learning, though the materials on the practice-based learning web site referred to earlier are helpful. On a more philosophical level the excellent and extensive materials on the Infed web site are highly recommended. Both addresses appear earlier in this chapter. On reflective practice:

Schön, D. (1983) *The Reflective Practitioner: How Professionals think in Action.* London: Basic Books. This is an accessible introduction.

Fraser, S. and Matthews, S. (2008) *The Critical Practitioner in Social Work and Health Care.* London: Sage/OU.

3

COLLECTING, SELECTING AND ASSESSING EVIDENCE AND INFORMATION: BECOMING RESEARCH AWARE

Graham Brotherton

SUMMARY CHAPTER CONTENTS

- Sources of information
- Finding research and information
- Evidence-based practice
- Approaches to research
- Research techniques
- Ethics of research

Learning objectives

By the end of this chapter, you should be able to:

- Identify a range of sources where health and social care information and research can be found.

- Evaluate published research in terms of its methodological appropriateness.

- Understand the idea of evidence-based practice in health and social care.

- Discuss ethical issues related to health and social care research.

Sources of information

In this section we will be considering how to find the information that you need in order to study effectively. There are a range of sources of information available to you, whether you are at work, in your college or university, or at home, especially if you have access to a computer. In this chapter we will look at some of the useful sources available to you and how to access them. We will also consider how to look critically at sources in order to judge the usefulness of what you find.

Workplace information

There are two sources of information within the workplace that are likely to be particularly helpful to you: policies and procedures; and the 'trade press'.

Policies and procedures are central to work in health and social care; they provide a framework for practice within any organisation, but they are also much more than this. They provide a way of looking at a broad range of issues. Policies in many areas are the practical application of government policy and as such they also reflect broader social values and attitudes. Evaluating organisational policies can give us considerable insight into these underpinning values and the way in which they influence the development of practice. The way in which policy at all levels is made is considered more fully in Chapter 6.

Activity

Look at the module structure for your particular programme and at the range of in-house policies your organisation has. Try to identify which policies may be useful to you at different stages on the course. If your setting is part of a larger organisation try to find out if there are policies with which you are not familiar (your manager/mentor/training officer might be able to help you locate appropriate polices).

Evaluating policies

The policies and procedures which exist in your organisation do not exist in isolation, they are influenced by a range of external factors. As you identify the key policies for your organisation try to find out what has influenced them. Some the key factors might include:

- Legislation, e.g. to comply with the National Health Service and Community Care Act 1990 or the Children Act 2004 or the codes of practice associated with legislation, such as the Special Educational Needs Code of Practice (DfES, 2001).
- Current views of good practice in terms of working with particular groups.

- Organisational values, e.g. the provision of services in a faith-based context.
- Financial or other resource constraints.

Each of these issues is explored more fully in the chapters in Section Two of this book.

The 'trade press'

Every sector has a range of magazines which are produced specifically for it. Within the health and social care sector there are a range of publications aimed at the sector in general or specific parts of it. These provide a very effective way of keeping up to date with current debates and issues. Among the most widely available are *Community Care* and the *Health Service Journal*. In addition there are magazines aimed at those working with particular groups, e.g. *Children Now* and *Mental Health Today*. The great advantage of the 'trade' press is that it is current, practice focused and usually produced in an accessible writing style. However, for higher education courses there are some limitations: articles are often fairly brief and make limited reference to research, they are usually written by professionals or others with a particular interest, and may not always give a full or objective overview of the issues. This is not to say that the trade press is not an important resource, but that it is important to use it as one of a range of sources.

It is also important to note that the 'broadsheet' general press also offers extensive coverage of health and social care issues. Of particular relevance is the *Society* supplement which is part of the *Guardian* on a Wednesday, which is an invaluable source of material (and contains a lot of relevant jobs!). It is worth making sure that at a fairly early stage you have a look at the range of 'trade' titles and broadsheets available in your setting and college/university library and try to identify which titles might be useful to you. You might also wish to purchase a broadsheet newspaper; student discounts are often available.

Using email updates

Many of the journals, newspapers and organisations referred to in this section offer the opportunity to subscribe to regular email-based updates which are usually free. These can be a very efficient way of staying up to date with current issues. One example is the Guardian Society briefing details which can be found on the paper's web site.

Online resources

Before moving on to consider many of the excellent resources available online it is worth reminding you about the excellent glossary of key health and social care terms available at the http://www.cpa.org.uk web site.

Academic gateways

A valuable and freely available resource, they differ from search engines such as Google in that they only search a range of resources that have been selected by academic librarians with subject knowledge. They can be accessed through www.intute.ac.uk, with the Social Science section being the most useful, though the Health and Life Sciences section is also very helpful.

Activity

Look at Intute and try to locate some resources which are useful to you. If you find it difficult and seem to be getting too many or too few resources, you might want to look at the activity on Boolean searching later in this chapter.

Subject gateways are catalogues of resources specifically aimed at the higher education community in particular areas. The most useful one for health and social care is the Social Work and Policy gateway which can be found at www.swap.ac.uk. There are, though, a number of other resources which might be useful and the full list of subject gateways can be found from the www.hecademy.ac.uk web site; the resources are of variable depth and quality but are well worth exploring.

The www.vts.intute.ac.uk page contains a list of Internet tutorials for higher education students. While there is not a general one for health and social care, there are several for related groups/areas, e.g. social work, nursing, social policy. They are all very easy to use as a starting point for the Internet research novice.

There is also a health and social care tutorial aimed at further education, which, although a little basic for study at this level, nonetheless contains lots of useful resources and a clear guide to using them.

> HANDY HINT
>
> For all the Intute tutorials, if you want to be able to access the web sites referred to in the tutorial while you are in the tutorial, click on links basket on the left-hand side of the page, then click on disable links basket on the next page. If you then want to save sites, you will need to use the favourites menu on your PC.

Government websites

Government websites provide probably the most comprehensive resource in terms of legislation, policy, research and practice guidance. However, the sheer size of some of the departmental web sites can make information hard to find. One way of dealing with this is to use the 'public face' of the government web sites, www.direct.gov.uk. However, not all information is available from here and it is sometimes more useful to go into the departmental web sites at the Department of Health (health and adult social care) www.dh.gov.uk, Department for Education and Skills (for children's services) www.dfes.gov.uk or for criminal-justice-related information the Home Office, www.homeoffice. gov.uk. All of these web sites have research sections containing details of government-funded research.

Research and policy organisations

There are a wide range of organisations which play a role on developing or influencing policy and practice. Those listed below are just a sample

- Joseph Rowntree Foundation, www.jrf.org.uk. One of the largest independent social research organisations with an emphasis on health and social care research. The 'findings' section provides excellent summaries of all the research that the foundation has commissioned.
- Sainsbury centre for Mental Health, www.scmh.org.uk. This provides access to a range of research on mental health issues, plus a lot of other useful material on these issues.
- The King's Fund, www.kingsfund.org.uk. This is a large health-related research and policy organisation.

'Think-tanks' are independent organisations with an emphasis on trying to influence policy. They are a useful source of information on current debates and thinking. There are think–tanks which operate from a variety of political perspectives and again this is only a sample (a full list can be found at http://www.policylibrary.com/uk/). Some of those with an active interest in health and social care policy include:

- Civitas, www.civitas.org.uk, a right of centre free market think-tank.
- Centre for Policy Studies, www.cps.org.uk, another free market think-tank.
- Institute for Public Policy Research, www.ippr.org.uk, a centre left think-tank.
- Demos, www.demos.co.uk, another centre/centre left think-tank.

(The terms free market and left and right are defined in Chapter 6.)

Specialist organisations

There are a range of organisations which produce information that relates to particular groups from both 'user' and 'professional' perspectives. The following are just a sample:

- Mind, www.mind.org.uk. A superb resource on mental health issues, in particular the fact sheets and briefings within the information section provide an excellent source of policy and practice information related to mental health.

- The Mental Health Foundation, www.mentalhealth.org.uk. Again a large and well-organised resource with a broad range of relevant information.
- Foundation for People with Learning Disabilities, www.learningdisabilities.org.uk. This foundation has a large and easy-to-use site with lots of useful information about learning disabilities.
- Mencap, www.mencap.org.uk. A good range of resources, especially in the publications section. Also includes some good examples of material designed to be accessible to people with a learning disability.
- Age Concern, www.ageconcern.org.uk. Another large and easy-to-use web site with a focus on older people's issues.
- Barnardo's, www.barnardos.org.uk. A range of resources for those working with children and families.

In addition to searching, utilising the subject gateways described earlier enables you to find organisations providing specialist information and support for particular groups of people who use health and social care services.

In looking at any of the materials described in this section it is important to bear in mind the need to read 'critically', which means thinking about the strengths and limitations of any source. It is not always easy to separate 'research' from 'policy' or even opinion. Practical ways of doing this are discussed in the reading research section below. Before considering how to 'look at' research, though, we need to look at why research is so central to good practice in health and social care.

Evidence-based practice

Gomm and Davies (2000) point out that government policy and professional guidance are increasingly calling for practice to be 'evidence based'. There is a need to justify the decisions that practitioners make that affect people's lives. This includes the need to develop an awareness of the scope and limitations of research through the use of critical appraisal skills.

While there are those who would argue that only certain types of research are appropriate for basing practice upon, e.g. the use of randomised control trials, or methods which approximate to this, it is not the intention to make this argument here. The suggestion here is that good practice evolves in a number of ways, but central to this is learning both from direct evaluations of practice and from more general research which is relevant to the setting or user group we are working with. Evidence-based practice is not simply about being able to make direct comparisons, but about having an awareness of and an open mind to changing views of good practice balanced with a healthy scepticism about whether these really stem from evidence.

What do we mean by evidence-based practice?

Evidence-based practice is about choosing the options that are most likely to lead to a good outcome for the people we work with. Or, to put it another way, using an evidence-based approach to practice will increase the likelihood that successful outcomes will occur (Centre for Evidence Based Social Services, 2004).

In other words, an evidence-based approach claims to be:
- Systematic – it attempts to be aware of the research which is around and how this is relevant to practice.
- Open – it attempts to look at evidence openly and assess the strengths and weaknesses on the basis of the 'case' that is made.
- Empowering – it enables service users to receive currently accepted 'good practice' in partnership with staff who are themselves able constructively to challenge practice.
- As such it is based on the effective use of research to support practice and requires practitioners to be able to find and evaluate research and policy/guidance.

Finding research

As suggested above, being able to read, evaluate and where appropriate recognise the practical implications of research is an important element of your studies. In order to do this, though, you need to be able to track down appropriate sources. This section looks at how to do this.

Many of the sources outlined at the start of this chapter are useful here, though in most cases they will only provide summaries of research. In addition there are a number of more explicitly research-focused sources. The first of these is refereed journals, which are often considered to be the 'gold standard' in that every article that is published has been read and evaluated by experts in the field and articles therefore represent an accurate and current contribution to knowledge in the specific area. It does need to be pointed out, however, that not all articles published in refereed journals are actually research reports.

There are a wide range of journals available and they can be accessed in three main ways. Firstly, directly from your college library – the library is likely to have a list of the journals which are taken. Secondly, it is often possible to access journals online; again access varies between institutions and your library should be able to provide you with a list of the journals you can access. Thirdly, you can often obtain copies of articles through interlibrary loan, though there is sometimes a charge for this; again your library will advise on the way things work in your institution.

It is also possible in some cases to access the journals kept by other higher education institutions and there are particular schemes that enable you to do this (see www.sconul.ac.uk for details). In order to make effective use of journal material, it is advisable to become familiar with the use of databases. Once again some of these are subscription based, so you will need to check which ones you have access to.

Using databases

Databases are collections of referenced material usually put together by librarians. Each one works slightly differently and you have to 'get inside the heads' of the people that put them together, in the sense of working out how material is categorised. The following tips can help with this:

- Keep a record of search terms used in each database and whether they generate data, so for example you might find that the term 'learning disability' works well in one database but in another you may have to use 'learning difficulty' or even in the case of some international databases, 'mental handicap'. Over time you begin to build up a picture of which terms work best in particular databases.
- Try to think creatively. You may as illustrated above have to think of a number of variations on a search term before you find much material. Using a thesaurus can be very helpful here.
- Become familiar with Boolean searching. This is a way of refining searches which helps you to find precisely the material you want. Most academic databases (and some web search engines) support Boolean searching, which is based around using key words or symbols to broaden or narrow searching.
- Keep a record of what worked in particular databases – it saves time for future searches.

Examples of useful databases

Web of Knowledge (wok.mimas.ac.uk) is one, but to access this you will need an 'Athens' password. Your library should be able to provide you with this. This is a massive database and you are likely to find the Social Science Citation Index the most useful section. As with all databases it can take a while to get used to. See tips on using databases below.

Another is http://www.scie-socialcareonline.org.uk/. This is a much more specifically social-care-focused database (as well as a range of other resources) which provides a very useful topic-based index, making it easy to search, though it may take a few attempts to work out what sort of information can be found in each topic category.

Boolean searching

To give some examples: AND (Boolean words are always written in capitals) or the +
symbol are used to combine terms, so 'mental health AND care' would include everything
which includes both terms. NOT (or -) excludes specific terms, so 'care NOT mental health'
would bring up material about care that does not refer to mental health. OR enables you
to search for more than one term, e.g. 'learning difficulties OR learning disabilities'. Most
databases have a help section which gives advice on using Boolean searching.

Your university or college librarians are also likely to be able to help.

Systematic reviews

Systematic reviews are an attempt to pull together all existing research/knowledge
on a particular topic or issue. Some adherents of evidence-based practice consider them to be the 'gold standard' in terms of evidence to support practice.
They attempt to identify, synthesise and analyse all of the literature on a particular topic and are based on the use of explicit criteria. In this way it is argued
that they reduce the potential problem of conscious or unconscious bias. They
emerged from quantitative research approaches and there are those who argue
that they are not always as appropriate or as easy to utilise when qualitative
studies are involved; this debate is considered more fully later in this chapter.
Nonetheless they do provide a useful starting point for taking stock of the evidence in relation to a particular area (assuming that you can find one which is
relevant to your interests). A useful way of at least beginning to search is to type
systematic review into the search box on the front page of Social Care Online
(the address is in the box on using databases later in this chapter). It has been
argued that systematic reviews are essential to improve the evidence base of
social care and in the development of best practice guidelines. While this view
can be challenged on methodological grounds, it is important for practitioners
to be aware of this increasingly important debate.

A range of health-related reviews (though some also have significant social
care content) can be found through http://www.phru.nhs.uk and some very
useful material (though primarily from the United States) can be found on the
Campbell Collaboration web site, http://www.campbellcollaboration.org/.

Reading research critically

With the increasing influence of evidence-based practice it is increasingly
important for practitioners to be able to read and evaluate published research.

Research is undertaken by a variety of agencies and for a variety of reasons, so it is vital to be able to assess the strength and weaknesses of the claims made by research. There are a number of useful questions which can form a basis for evaluating research (and other academic writing):

- Who wrote this? Is the research being undertaken by an individual/organisation that has particular expertise in the area? Has it been undertaken by someone approaching the research from a particular political/ideological/professional perspective?
- Why? Is it promoting a particular approach (or even a good or service)?
- For what reason? Is it making a claim for resources? Is it 'pure' research (if it is possible to do pure research)?
- When? How recent is the material? Has policy or practice changed since the research was undertaken/material was written?
- Where was the research carried out? Does the social/cultural context of the research enable it to be used appropriately in the context you are thinking of using it, e.g. can American research always be easily applied to the UK context?
- Who was involved?
- Where is the research being reported? Is the research in a refereed journal? If not, is it being summarised? Can you be confident that the summary gives a clear overall picture?
- Was the method appropriate to justify the claims being made? (This is discussed more fully in the next section.) Does it seem to you that the method used would give the sort of findings/information being presented?
- How convinced are you by the evidence? What is your 'gut feeling' about the research? Why do you think this is?

Gathering information directly

As you read this section you might find the following web sites particularly helpful: The excellent web site Research Mindedness in Social Work and Social care at http://www.resmind.swap.ac.uk gives lots of useful information on many of the topics discussed. The 'Are you Research Minded?' quiz is a good place to start. There is an excellent glossary of common research terms and their meaning via http://www.whatworksforchildren.org.uk.

As suggested previously, there is an increasing emphasis in health and social care practice on the need for evidence to support good practice. This happens on at least two levels, firstly as an element of quality assurance and inspection systems (discussed more fully in Chapter 6 in terms of process and Chapter 10 in terms of practice implications) and secondly as a way of developing good practices. It is this second level which will be the focus of this chapter, though it must be made clear that there is of course considerable overlap between the two levels.

Activity

Think of the way in which information about the service you provide is collected.

- o   Who collects it?
- o   How is it collected?
- o   How is it used?
- o   Would you describe this as research? Why or why not?

We gather information in a variety of ways, e.g. as part of the assessment and care planning process and of monitoring its implementation, through satisfaction surveys and other forms of user feedback, as well as in putting together information for inspection and informally through conversations with colleagues and service users. In doing this we are often seeking to evaluate the appropriateness and effectiveness of what we are doing. In this section we will be considering how we can make these judgements on the basis of evidence and some of the problems in deciding what constitutes 'good' evidence.

In order to gather evidence in a systematic and reliable way, we become involved in a process of research. For something to be called research we often think of its being gathered in a formal way and usually in order to address some pre-set question or problem (though this definition is not without its limitations). 'Experts' often from the academic community are often called upon to undertake research of this kind. There is, though, a tradition within the health and social care community (and in related areas such as education) of research undertaken by practitioners in order to address workplace problems, usually referred to as action research, and this chapter will include a discussion of both approaches. In addition, as stated previously we often gather information for other purposes but do so in a systematic way and use it for 'official' purposes, e.g. an audit. We do need therefore to be aware of the strengths and limitations of the various approaches to gathering 'data'. In this chapter 'data' will be used to refer to anything gathered in a structured way, whether this is qualitative or quantitative information.

Qualitative versus quantitative approaches

There are broadly two approaches to social research, which stem from different approaches to how we can obtain and interpret information. Quantitative research, sometimes (and perhaps over-simply) called 'scientific' research, is concerned with obtaining measurable data, often for the purposes of comparison or statistical analysis. It is concerned with obtaining factual information in an objective and value-free way, which can then be used to develop models that can be tested in subsequent research in order to check their robustness. The basis of this approach is a set of ideas usually referred to as positivism, which suggest that true knowledge can only be obtained by scientific approaches and that research should focus upon that which can be directly observed. This can be contrasted with qualitative approaches, which are concerned with attitude and perception. They are concerned with how people make sense of the world around them and are less concerned with notions of neutrality and objectivity, highlighting that all researchers have preconceptions and values which will influence their approach. There is not time here to develop the arguments about the philosophical foundations of research, but there are a number of excellent introductory research books around which are listed in the further reading section.

In recent years in health and social care research there has been a move towards using 'mixed methods' which often combine elements of both qualitative and quantitative research. One of the justifications for this is the idea of *triangulation*. This suggests that by using a variety of methods it is possible to check whether there is correspondence between the different sorts of data being collected and thereby gain a fuller picture, thus increasing the validity of the research. It has to be noted, though, that triangulation between methods is complex in practice and that caution needs to be exercised when attempting to use triangulation to make more general claims for any piece of research.

Two terms which you will often come across in research are reliability and validity and it may be useful to define them here. *Reliability* is concerned with whether the results would be replicated by using the same instrument/ approach in the same circumstances. *Validity* is concerned with whether the research can be said to be presenting an accurate picture of the area being researched. Both terms are subject to some debate and are somewhat problematic in practice, especially in relation to qualitative data. (At a very simple level can research about opinion or perception ever be truly reliable or valid? But does that mean it is not important to carry out this sort of research?) However, they remain important concepts which need to be considered fully in research design, reporting and evaluation.

The key issue is that when undertaking any form of research, no matter how informal, it is crucial to be aware of the strengths and limitations of any chosen approach and the implications that this has both for the nature of any findings and for any conclusions which can be drawn. Some research will inevitably be more tentative, especially if dealing with for example complex issues of practice, or issues around service users' attitudes or perceptions. This does not mean that these are not areas worthy of investigation, just that care needs to be taken in the way they are interpreted.

Within the context of all research it is important to note that a central consideration is that of appropriateness: it is not that one research method is right and another is wrong, but that different approaches generate differing kinds of information. The judgement of research needs therefore has to be based on a consideration of whether the research was of the 'right' kind to generate the sort of information which would answer the questions the researcher was asking.

Activity

You want to investigate the 'satisfaction' of service users with the services you offer. What would be the advantages and disadvantages of using: (a) questionnaires; (b) interviews? (Assume for the purpose of this exercise that your service users would be able to contribute effectively using either approach.)

Comment: It depends. Questionnaires (see next section) are easy to administer and easy to collate but in most cases give you only superficial information. For example, on a form produced by one health organisation patients were asked whether they were not satisfied, satisfied or very satisfied with the service they had received. How can we judge how people distinguished between the latter two categories, and does it really matter, given that both indicate satisfaction?

However, if we want in-depth information, talking to people at length about their experiences is likely to generate much richer information, but information which is harder to collate in a simple form. Gathering information in this way is also much more time consuming.

As suggested previously, the key question here is appropriateness: why are we gathering information? What do we want to use it for? If we are simply monitoring ongoing satisfaction at a particular setting or with a particular service, then it may be that a questionnaire is the most appropriate. However, if we want to reform or develop services it may be more useful to gather information through interviews.

Techniques of research in health and social care

Action research

As referred to previously, a particular approach, which has been widely used in health, care and educational settings, is action research. Action research has been defined as 'a form of research carried out by practitioners into their own practices' (Smith, 2001; cites Kemmis and Carr, 1986). It is therefore explicitly work related and linked to notions of developing good practice. The full process of action research is to identify a work-related problem or issue, to gather information about the problem or issue, to identify collaboratively a strategy for 'solving' the problem or issue and then to implement and monitor the strategy. Where appropriate this can prove to be the starting point for another cycle of action research. In practice many action research projects (especially those undertaken as student projects!) only go as far as identifying issues that can subsequently be used as a basis for developing/improving practice. It can of course be argued that this is not genuinely action research, though it does provide an introduction to the approach. A good summary of approaches to and some of the problems with action research can be found through http://www.infed.org.

Before looking at particular techniques it is important to point out that these are different to approaches. Particular techniques may be used within either of the broad philosophical approaches outlined earlier; for example, a survey (see below) could be either qualitative or quantitative in approach depending upon the way in which it is designed (or even contain elements of both). It is therefore crucial that any research instrument is designed in such a way that the researcher is clear about what kind of data is being collected as this obviously has significant implications for how any data should be analysed.

Particular techniques of data collection will now be outlined.

Surveys

Surveys are pieces of research which attempt to look at a representative sample of a particular 'population'. This can mean a specific population, the patients of a hospital, the users of a day service or the population as a whole. Because many populations are too large to involve everyone, in most cases a sample is used. Samples can be either *representative*, i.e. designed to reflect the population as a whole, or *opportunistic*, i.e. assembled from those who are available to the researcher. Samples become important if we are claiming that the research gives an accurate picture of the whole population we are seeking to research. This can only be genuinely claimed if we can demonstrate that our sample was of the representative kind. There are various ways of doing this and where this is likely to be an issue you are strongly advised to read a more specialised text. There is a very good introduction to the issues in Robson (2002). It is of course important to point out that being representative in this general sense may not be important for small workplace-based projects as by definition these are perhaps better considered as case studies.

Interviews

Interviews are widely used in health and social research, but there can of course be difficulties in using them with those groups of service users who may find it more difficult to articulate their thoughts, though multiple communication systems, e.g. speech plus some form of physical or symbolic communication, have been used to try to minimise the impact of this. While interviews offer a valuable research tool, there are several important factors which need to be considered. Firstly, issues of design. There are three broad types of interview: structured, where set questions are used; semi-structured, where a loose list of questions/prompts are used as a basis for a conversation; and unstructured, where there are no pre-set questions or prompts. Each has advantages and disadvantages:

- Structured interviews are easy to compare and collate afterwards, but can be stilted to do and may lead to important information not being collected if any area is omitted from the schedule. They are also highly researcher lead.
- Unstructured interviews have the opposite problems. They are much more likely to lead to rich information, but they are difficult to collate and difficult (if not impossible) to do for inexperienced (and possibly most other!) researchers.
- Semi-structured interviews offer a methodological compromise, with a loose structure to provide researchers with a framework, but also the opportunity to let the interview flow into a variety of areas. They do still pose problems of comparability and collation.

Observations

Observations have been widely used in research with young children, but have a useful role to play in health and social care research. Again there are two broad categories:

- Unstructured observations, in which an attempt is made to capture as much information as possible about the whole of a situation.
- Structured observations, in which a decision is taken in advance to focus primarily on a particular range of features or issues, using some form of schedule or checklist.

As with interviews there are advantages and disadvantages to both techniques. Structured techniques (assuming they are undertaken appropriately) give a clear picture of a limited range of activity. Unstructured techniques give a fuller picture but run the risk of missing key details in trying to gain a broad picture; similar issues also apply on terms of collating and analysing data to those described for interviews above.

Questionnaires

Questionnaires are a widely used technique, which enables a large amount of data to be gathered reasonably efficiently. There are, though, both practical and methodological problems. The main practical problem is response rates. Questionnaires are notoriously difficult to achieve good response rates on, especially if they are administered indirectly. Postal questionnaires are particularly difficult to get returned and if you intend to use them, this needs to be built into the way in which any research is designed. Unless you have some way of ensuring a higher return rate it may be wise to plan around a response rate of around one-third for any form of questionnaire.

On a broader level particular attention needs to be paid to how questions are designed; there is no opportunity to ask for clarification or to develop points afterwards, so questionnaires are a 'one-shot' approach. It is important then to think carefully about wording. Bell (2005) includes a chapter which gives a clear and comprehensive guide to the practicalities of questionnaire research. The issue of sampling is particularly important in questionnaire research, especially if you wish to make any general claims based on your results.

Life story or narrative research

Life story or narrative research has been used very effectively, especially in social care research. This is a fairly specialised technique which often uses repeat interviews plus documentary research or photographs with a view to building up a picture of someone's personal history. It can be useful for understanding how and why people come to be users of care services and is also claimed by some people to have direct therapeutic benefits. This is an under-utilised approach but requires very careful planning and careful consideration of its appropriateness in terms of working with particular individuals or groups.

Case study research

Case studies are pieces of research which look in depth at a specific 'case', sometimes for an individual or group of people and sometimes for a specific setting, e.g. a residential home or a social work office. The purpose of case study research is to examine a particular 'instance' in a lot of detail. As a result it is always difficult to generalise from case study research, though its strength is that it gives insight into one situation which may be transferable into others. Case studies can also give useful 'pointers' for possible research into similar settings. When using case studies it is important to ensure that you are clear about the 'boundaries' of a case (i.e. are you researching all of a setting or a particular subset, e.g. a 'ward', 'unit' or particular group of people who use the service, as this again has implications for data analysis?). Case studies are not in themselves a research technique so data collection will need to utilise one or more of the other methods as described in this section.

Comparative research

Another commonly used approach is to compare aspects of practice within health and social care settings as a way of emphasising similarities and differences and possible explanations of factors which influence this. This often takes the form of case studies of more than one setting. It is an approach which is potentially extremely useful but needs careful planning in terms of ensuring that the chosen 'cases' allow for meaningful comparison and discussion.

Documentary analysis

Most agencies in the health and social care sector produce a range of internal documents. These vary from policy documents to internal reports and position papers (see Chapter 6). They provide a very useful resource in terms of undertaking research, but need to be used carefully. The key questions for reading research later in this chapter can provide a framework for doing this. There is also a very helpful chapter in Denscombe (2003) the full reference for which can be found in the section on further reading.

The ethics of research in health and social care settings

A key issue in all health and social care research is that of ethics. In some senses research ethics should be a straightforward issue in an area where there is a constant emphasis on the concept of ethical practice. If something can be considered good practice in health and social care terms, it is likely to be an ethical approach in research terms. Ethics can be defined in a number of ways which are discussed more fully in Chapter 5. One useful checklist for looking at ethical issues in the research context is presented in the box here:

Informed consent: Are all participants aware of the purpose of the research and what their own role within it will be?

Openness and honesty: Is the research being conducted in a transparent manner? That is, are all participants able to find out how their contribution 'fits' into the bigger picture and if appropriate to challenge any assumptions made?

Protection from harm: What steps have been taken to ensure that participants are not harmed by participation, e.g. by being exposed to inappropriate questions?

The right to withdraw: Are all participants clear that they do not have to take part and that if they do decide to withdraw from the research that data relating to them will be removed from the research?

Confidentiality: What steps have been taken to ensure that all data is stored and used in a way which does not allow the identification of any of the agencies or individuals involved?

(Continued)

(Continued)

***Debriefing*:** Are all participants able to access copies of findings etc. if they wish to?

***Compliance with institutional and professional codes of practice*:** Many health and care agencies have organisational codes of practice and may in some cases require that any research undertaken complies with these. Have you taken appropriate action to investigate and if necessary comply with these?

'Doing' research

As a teacher supervising research projects at a variety of levels over a number of years, by far the commonest problems that I have encountered is a lack of clarity about what is being researched. Crucial to any piece of research in the workplace or elsewhere is being clear about what you are trying to find out. It is therefore vital to have a research question or questions, which fulfil two central criteria:

- It/they must be precise in terms of what you are seeking to investigate.
- It must be possible actually to answer the question/s through the research and using the chosen methods (sometimes referred to as 'operationalisation').

Activity

Think back to the activity earlier in this chapter. Imagine you want to investigate how satisfied a group of older people are with the home care that they receive. How could you 'operationalise' this?

While there are clearly a number of ways in which this could be approached, the central issue is how do we make sense of 'satisfaction', as this could mean a number of different things? For example, for one person this might simply mean how well the various tasks that they require assistance with are undertaken, for someone else the key feature may be the quality of the interaction with the home carer, and for others it may be a balance between the two or indeed a range of other factors, e.g. how flexible the worker is etc.

None of these could be said to be 'right' or 'wrong' definitions of satisfaction but any piece of research needs to be clear about which single or multiple definition(s) of 'satisfaction' it is using and the consequences that this might have in terms of both the design and ultimate usefulness of the research.

Involving service users in research

As practice in health and social care has changed to take greater account of the views of service users, there has also been increasing interest in involving service users in all stages of the research process as active participants and partners rather than as passive subjects. Obviously the issues involved will vary from group to group and there are considerable differences in the issues around working with, for example, young children as opposed to mental health service users. A number of organisations have developed ethical codes which specifically address the issues of service user involvement (e.g. the Social Research Association, www.the-sra.org.uk). While there may be some ethical and practical issues that do need to be addressed, the arguments for involving those who use services are so strong in terms of good practice that there is an urgent need for more research of this type.

SUMMARY

This chapter has considered the key area of finding and using information and research. In attempting to summarise such a broad range of information a couple of key points are worth highlighting. Firstly, there are a range of useful sources which are easily accessible to you in the workplace and elsewhere but it is important to read critically: do not take research or other writing at face value but try to think about factors such as perspective and appropriateness of method as discussed in this chapter. Secondly, it is important to recognise the increasing importance of evidence-based practice, but once again to engage with this in a positive but critical way.

Review questions   ?

- What is meant by evidence-based practice in health and social care?
- What are the main approaches and techniques of social research and what are the strengths and weaknesses of each?
- Where should you look to find relevant research for your course or setting?

Further reading

Bell, J. (2005) *Doing your research project: a guide for first-time researchers in education,* 4th edn. Buckingham: Open University Press. Though education focused this is an accessible introduction with an invaluable chapter on questionnaires.

Blaxter, L. et al. (2001) *How to Research,* 2nd edn. Maidenhead: Open University Press. A clear and accessible introduction to research for first-time researchers.

Bryman, A. (2001) *Social Research Methods.* Oxford: Oxford University Press. Contains a more detailed discussion of the issues.

Denscombe, M. (2003) *The Good Research Guide,* 2nd edn. Maidenhead: Open University Press. Another clear and helpful text – especially in terms of the practicalities of research.

Gomm, R. and Davies, C. (eds) (2000) *Using Evidence in Health and Social Care.* London: Sage. Gives a clear overview of the evidence-based practice debate.

Robson, C. (2002) *Real World Research.* London: Blackwell. Another accessible and helpful text.

SECTION TWO

Theory and Practice

4 THE SOCIAL CONTEXT OF HEALTH AND SOCIAL CARE

Robert Mears

SUMMARY CHAPTER CONTENTS

- UK government expenditure on heath and social care and the 'mixed economy of care'
- The challenges to medicine from critics
- Health inequalities
- Acute and chronic illness
- Stigma
- Future social and cultural change and the challenges posed to the relationships between health and social care professionals

---

Learning objectives

By the end of this chapter, you should be able to:

- Understand what is meant by the 'social context' of health and the ways in which social structure impacts upon health.

- See how sociological theory and evidence help to clarify some of the dominant issues in health and social care.

- Describe some of the contested areas in health and social care and be able to make some contribution to these debates.

Introduction

Wherever health and social care work takes place, in hospital, hospice, residential institution or in the home, it is important to understand that beyond a particular encounter there is always a wider social context. This 'social context' can include the wider social determinants of health, prevailing epidemiological trends and the characteristics of the groups delivering and receiving care. What happens in health and social care takes place in a context which embraces social values and attitudes, economic decisions, political priorities and cultural beliefs. 'Caring' is usually a meeting between people who are likely to differ in terms of age, ethnic group, social class, religious affiliation, economic power, and so on. Critically, it will also involve relationships between people with varying levels of dependence and independence. The challenge of this chapter is to set the 'caring' relationship in this wider social context.

The connections between the 'individual' and the 'social' were explored by the American sociologist, C. Wright Mills. He argued that the sociological imagination involved the ability to make connections between individual troubles and broader social processes. This way of thinking is not typical because, 'In Western industrial societies the ethic of individualism has led to a concentration on the position and activities of the individual and to individualistic explanations. People have not perceived the regularities in the patterns of social behaviour but only the individual differences' (Hurd, 1974: 6). This chapter introduces the idea that many aspects of health and social care can best be explained when we understand more about these prevailing patterns. Care does not take place in a vacuum but is shaped by social, cultural, political and economic factors.

A starting point is some grasp of the sheer scale of government investment in health and social care. It is obvious that the wider society, in the shape of government decisions about resource allocation, is critical. Government policy will determine not just how much is spent but how it is spent. There will always be tension around the allocation of scarce resources. Government policies also help shape decisions about the most appropriate place for the delivery of care – home or institution. In 2007–8 total UK government public spending will be around £580 billion. This is over £9000 for every man woman and child in the UK and health and social care and social protection takes up nearly half of this. Around £146 billion goes on pensions, invalidity benefit, support for the unemployed, etc., £90 billion on the NHS and £23 billion on personal social services (HM Treasury, 2006). It is obvious that such sums cannot be allocated without a wider debate about value for money, affordability, entitlement and what economists refer to as 'opportunity costs' – how those resources might have been spent differently. So, 'formal' health and social care is usually paid for by governments and delivered by state employees. State expenditure is often supplemented by private spending and contributions made by voluntary agencies and charities. It is usual for care to be delivered by a mixture of the public, private and voluntary sector, and what family friends and neighbours provide informally. The particular balance between 'formal' and 'informal' provision is always a matter of policy debate and is likely to shift over time for particular individuals and will depend, partly, on what kinds of political choices are made by the wider society.

It is useful to make this distinction between the formal system of care provided by doctors, nurses, social workers, therapists, etc., who provide some kind of professional service, and the informal care advice and support provided by friends, neighbours and family members, so-called lay care. For most of human history lay care was all that was available. It is only in the last century or so in rich countries that the balance of care has shifted in the direction of state-provided 'formal' health and social care. It is important for professionals to understand the changing balance between professional and lay care and the ways in which these are related. There is also a growing possibility of conflict between formal and informal carers. Lay people and professionals may have different (incompatible) beliefs about what is the best course of action and they may have different opinions of the role of the person cared for in decision making.

'Choice' implies priorities and this means politics. Professionals in health and social care may think of politics as little to do with their work. The word usually conjures up images of political parties and voting, and the decisions taken and policies adopted by councillors, MPs and governments. For social scientists, politics means the study of the distribution of power between and among individuals or groups. Power is an inevitable feature of all social relationships whether that is between two people in a marriage through to the relations between powerful nation-states. In this sense there are power relations between parents and children, carers and the cared, professionals and lay people. Max Weber argued that 'power can emerge from social relations in a drawing room as well as in the market, from the rostrum of a lecture hall as well as the command post of a regiment, from an erotic or charitable relationship as well as from scholarly discussion or athletics' (Weber, cited in O'Donnell, 1987: 512).

Politics can also refer to the value system that underpins our actions. It refers to the whole cluster of ideas that characterise what people think and feel we 'ought' to do. This raises important questions of duty, obligation and the 'appropriate' ways of responding to social problems or social need. Politics also encompasses the ideological options we choose. For example, once we say that something *ought* to be done, or there *ought* to be more spent on a particular group, we reveal our ideological choices. In the world of health and social care this can cover a wide range of choices – who pays for services, who 'ought' to deliver them, and what is the balance between, say, care in an institution and home care.

Activity

- o Choose an area of health and social care with which you are familiar and identify the mix of provision in this area.
- o Consider whether this area of health and social care is currently a political/ institutional priority – is the provision diminishing, stable or increasing?
- o Consider how it has been/is being shaped by economic, cultural and other factors.

To grasp the scale of demand, present and future, on formal and informal health carers, we need to understand the patterns of fertility and mortality that shape the demography of a society. The likely demand for care, at either end of the life cycle, is affected by the age structure of the population and the relative balance of old and young people. The UK, in common with most wealthy countries, has a falling fertility rate and a falling mortality rate. This gives us the distinctive feature of an ageing population with, in the UK, more people over 60 than under 16. This has triggered widespread debate about the costs and other consequences of an ageing society with economists and social policy analysts articulating concerns about the 'dependency ratio'. This refers to the relationship between the economically active and the 'dependent' population of the elderly, the sick and disabled, children, students and people at home caring for others. In policy circles this is a pressing issue, as witnessed by disputes about state retirement pensions and the viability of other welfare payments.

Making sense of 'care'

Because of an ageing population and the rise of chronic illness, more people are involved in paid and unpaid care of others than in the past. In addition to around 2 million employees of the NHS and social services, around 5.2 million people were providing unpaid care in England and Wales in 2003 and 2.8 million of these are over 50 (Office for National Statistics web site). Unsurprisingly a greater proportion of women than men were carers, both in the population as a whole and in age groups up to 64 years. The men who care are very likely to be caring for wives, while women are caring for husbands, children, parents and others. The proportion of adults providing care does vary substantially across the country. The local authorities with the highest rates of limiting long-term illness or disability had as much as 17 per cent of adults providing care to others.

'Care' is a simple four letter word. What could be easier to understand and explain? Yet it elicits a host of different and sometimes incompatible emotions. It can be carried out for love, duty, payment, guilt or some other sense of obligation. In reality more than one of these feelings can co-exist. The different meanings of the word have been carefully analysed by Carol Thomas. She deconstructs care into seven dimensions covering:

- identity of carer;
- identity of cared for;
- the interpersonal relationship between them;
- the nature of the care;
- the social domain (private/domestic);
- the economic relationship;
- and the institutional setting, e.g. home, residential setting, hospital, nursery, etc. (Thomas, 1993)

Activity

Take an example of 'caring' and analyse it using the seven dimensions outlined by Carol Thomas.

  Think of examples of the last time you carried out 'care' of another. What was the dominant motive for doing it? What emotions did it elicit?

Among 50 to 64 year olds, a greater proportion of women than men provide unpaid care, and a higher proportion provide intensive care (50 or more hours a week). The majority of older people continue to live in the community well into later life. Even when we look at the data for people aged over 90, around three-quarters were living in private households (Office for National Statistics web site). One measure of domestic support for people is the amount of home help provided by local authorities. The number of home help hours purchased or provided by councils in England has increased significantly over the past two decades. In 1994 it was 2.2 million hours but by 2004 this had risen to an estimated 3.4 million hours provided to around 355,600 households. While the overall number of hours supplied has increased, the number of households receiving council-funded home care services has fallen consistently since 1994. This suggests that councils are providing more intensive services for a smaller number of households (ONS web site).

Medicalisation

For much of the twentieth century the actions of health and social care professionals were usually seen in a positive light. Doctors and nurses in particular tended to be rated highly in any survey of public opinion and the value of their work was such that they enjoyed high levels of esteem. Indeed health services were generally seen as a 'good thing' and the public seemed to want higher levels of spending. Academic critics took a much more sceptical approach about the role of medicine in prolonging life and promoting health. Firstly, it was argued by McKeown (1976) that the contribution of medicine in conquering infectious disease and prolonging life has been exaggerated. He analysed falling death rates in England and Wales for infectious diseases after 1870 and claimed this had much more to do with improvements in nutrition, housing, sanitation and town and city planning (such as rubbish collection and clean air) and family limitation. Medical discoveries and treatments were insignificant because they were ineffective, harmful or appear when the death rates are already in decline. Other critics complained about a growing disillusion with medicine because of the escalating costs of health services with disappointing returns from investment in medical cures and treatments (Abel-Smith, 1996). Research showed that medical interventions were of limited benefit and that for many treatments there was little evidence of their effectiveness (Cochrane, 1972). In 2006 Professor Ian Roberts claimed that many emergency treatments for trauma in hospital A&E departments were of dubious benefit. He was quoted in a newspaper report saying that treatments had not been properly evaluated: 'If you have an injury you will be exposed to treatments that we really don't know whether they will do more harm than good.' After decades of use there was little or no hard evidence for the treatments' effectiveness. In 2004 Roberts published a study in the *Lancet* exposing the dangers of corticosteroids, used to reduce brain inflammation. Rather than improving the patients' condition it actually increased their chances of dying. The *Lancet* estimated that 10,000 people had been killed worldwide by the treatment in the 1980s and before. It is now rarely used in the UK (*Guardian*, 7 September 2006).

In addition the long-term, chronic 'diseases of affluence' turned out to be difficult to cure. The consequences of high-technology medicine also came to be seen in a more negative light and the doctor/patient relationship was seen as beset with problems. Even more radical was the claim that the medical profession was guilty of extending its power into areas of human life that should not concern it, and that many medical interventions were harmful, either because they led to further complications (such as drug side effects) or because they weakened the ability of people to manage their own lives (Illich, 1976). The critics argued that medical professionals claimed jurisdiction over wider areas of human life. Matters that might once have been the responsibility of priests, teachers, social workers or philosophers come to be seen as 'medical'. This starts a process of labelling something as a 'disease' and developing treatments that are managed and controlled by doctors. The critics argued that this made people unnecessarily dependent on the medical profession. For example, debates about adolescent sexuality, control of contraception and access to abortion became dominated by medical professionals when they are actually ethical issues. So-called 'natural' conditions such as childbirth, adolescence, ageing and death gradually became medicalised so that medical solutions become dominant. In recent times, childhood behaviour, sexual dysfunction, unhappiness, obesity and even shyness have become 'medicalised', with associated medical diagnosis, therapies and drug regimes. For Illich and other critics, this had the deleterious consequences of strengthening the power of the professionals at the expense of the ability of lay people to control their own bodies and their lives.

What is incontrovertible is the ever-rising demand for more health services. Most measures show a rise in demand for GP and hospital services of every kind. In England, for instance, the number of prescriptions issued by the NHS (excluding hospital prescriptions) has increased from an average of eight per person in 1989 to 12.5 in 2002 – an increase of 56 per cent. This is 'more than one prescription per month on average for every year of a person's life' (Busfield 2006: 297). Busfield claims that the pharmaceutical industry, in alliance with medicine,

> is shaping the ways in which society responds to a very broad range of problems. It is con-tributing to an extension of the territory of medical problems and the tendency to respond to problems by pill taking as if the problem will be solved by magic. This response often fails to grapple with the sources of these problems ... drugs provide an individualized solution to problems that often have social or structural origins, which are not tackled by pharmaceu-tical remedies. (2006: 310)

The critics of the growth of modern medicine claim then that we invest more of our resources into health care, demand more consultations, more treatments and more drugs without evidence of any real improvements in human health or happiness.

Activity

Give two examples of behaviour that has become medicalised in recent times.
  Are we becoming over-dependent on medical services?
  What are the alternatives to 'medicalisation'?

Health inequalities

There is a long history of research which shows the link between socio-economic position and health measured in life expectancy and sickness. The assumption of much of this work is that people who share a common economic position, with similar sources of wealth and power, will have similar life-chances. This view of 'life-chances' sees a person's health status as a sign of their past social position and, 'through the structured nature of social processes, as liable to selective accumulation of future advantage or disadvan-tage' (Blane, cited in Nettleton, 2006: 186). In other words, lifelong inequalities impact on the chances of being ill and dying young or old. Although the class structure is in flux, there is robust research evidence that establishes a strong and enduring link between socio-economic status and disease. Ever since data has been recorded on death certificates it was clear that occupation is linked to life expectancy. In the UK people in the lowest social class (5) can expect, on average, to live around nine years fewer than those in social class 1, the professional and managerial occupations. There are also marked inequalities of gender, region and minority ethnic group. Low socio-economic status is linked with 14 of the major cause-of-death categories in the International Classification of Diseases as well as many major psychological disorders. A recent survey showed that men in the most disadvantaged circumstances had more than double the mortality risk of men of the same age in the most advantaged circumstances (White et al., 2005). Research over many decades 'clearly establishes a strong and pervasive association between social conditions and disease' (Link and Phelan, 1995: 82).

Establishing that health inequalities exist does not tell us what causes them or what, if anything, could or should be done about them. Competing explanations include so-called structural and cultural explanations (Mears, 1992).

Structural explanations emphasise the material advantages and disadvantages of different socio-economic groups. The unequal distribution of resources – money, property, power, knowledge, status, etc. – is replicated in the distribution of health. One of the reasons for such persistent associations between economic position and ill-health is the fact that access to resources helps people avoid risks to health or to minimise the consequences of disease once it occurs.

Cultural explanations concentrate on the beliefs and behaviours of different groups, so-called 'lifestyle' factors.

There are also differences in people's access to what sociologists call 'social capital'. The American sociologist Robert Putnam defines it thus: 'social capital refers to connections among individuals – social networks and the norms of reciprocity and trustworthiness that arise from them' (Putnam, 2000: 19). The degree of social support enjoyed by people and the extent and quality of their social networks are seen as critical in understanding health status and coping with the consequences of disease. This idea of the beneficial health effects of strong social networks has generated a great deal of research recently. It has been shown that the extent and quality of social relationships – how strongly we are bonded to others – can have powerful influences on physical and mental health. In addition there are health consequences that arise from living in societies that are relatively unequal in terms of the wider distribution of wealth and opportunity (Wilkinson, 2000).

It may challenge 'common sense', but there is widespread agreement among researchers that expenditure on health services makes very little difference in terms of health outcomes. According to a recent review of the international data, 'beyond a certain threshold of expenditure, long since surpassed by most industrialized countries, one would be hard-pressed to conclude that spending more on health care leads to better health for a population' (Lewis et al., 2000:

510). Many of those concerned with health inequalities have argued that most effective steps that could be taken to prevent ill-health would probably not involve medical expertise at all because the determinants of ill-health are rooted in economic and social structure.

Activity

Why should health inequalities concern health and social care professionals?
   What measures do you suggest might be taken to address these inequalities?
   Is this a matter for central government only?

There are also controversial debates about the extent to which social class inequalities of health are narrowing or getting worse, and why it matters. It has been argued that they matter for three reasons. Firstly, how long we live and how sick we are is the ultimate measure of wider trends in socio-economic inequality. 'The size of our car or the desirability of our house and the number and type of exotic holidays are all a consequence of socio-economic inequalities. But none are as potent as life and death' (Carr-Hill, 1987: 87). Secondly, health inequalities provide a guide as to how effective health and social welfare services are. The persistence of such inequalities is a negative commentary on decades of 'free' health care and a welfare state. A third reason is to guide policy decisions so that we have a better idea of where to direct resources so they have maximum impact. Blaxter (2004) argues that inequalities at the start of life may be particularly controversial: 'It would appear that we have some feeling that that variability becomes inevitable with time, but at least there "ought" to be as much equality as possible at the start of life' (2004: 5).

Link and Phelan (1995) claim not only that health is affected by socio-economic status, gender and ethnicity, but that stressful life events of a social nature (e.g. the death of a loved one, loss of a job, or being a victim of crime) are implicated. The impact of such stressful life events can be mediated by the level of social support enjoyed by people, but it is clear that there are marked differences in the levels of social support enjoyed by different groups. It is often claimed that men and women, for example, can draw on different types of social support and 'having social support is generally associated with better health – but appears to be more important in shaping women's health' (Payne, 2006: 53).

Women and health

The improvements in life expectancy in the twentieth century have impacted on men and women differently. In the UK, life expectancy is higher for women than for men. In 2001 female life expectancy at birth was 80.4 years compared with 75.7 years for men. Although this seems like good news for women, the gap between men and women is smaller in terms of the number of years they can expect to live in good health, and women consistently report slightly higher rates of limiting and long-standing illnesses than men. In addition, 'Women of all ages report more use of GP and outpatient health services ... and women report higher levels of psychiatric morbidity' (Baggott, 2004: 25). As well as obvious bio-logical differences between men and women which account for gender differ-ences in health, sociological research has focused on material factors (levels of pay and pensions etc.) and social roles and relationships. The gender gap in terms of ageing and care is marked with, currently, more older, disabled women, and many are reduced to poverty in later life (Arber and Cooper, 2000). A key dif-ference – and an example of 'social context' – is that generational changes may be very important. Older women are less likely to have had a lifelong career and less likely to have enjoyed further or higher education. Just a couple of generations ago women were a tiny minority in many of the better paid and more prestigious professions. The relative poverty of older women today is partly, then, a conse-quence of lifelong exclusion from careers which makes them much more likely to be dependent on benefits and state pensions.

The dominant picture of men's and women's health has been that men die earlier but women are sicker! Researchers are now a little sceptical about this simplistic claim. According to Payne:

> this conventional wisdom has been challenged by research which suggests that variations in patterns of ill-health between men and women are rather more complex. Studies explor-ing the health of men and women have reported a narrower gap than before, with little evidence that women suffer more health problems overall during their lives. (2006: 9)

The changing social roles of men and women also impact on mortality levels and morbidity rates. Social and cultural changes have an impact on lifestyles. As younger women have enjoyed greater economic independence and cultural freedom, consumption of alcohol and tobacco has increased and women are more likely to suffer from eating disorders. So some social and cultural changes may confront women with greater health risks.

Typically, men are more likely to engage in risky behaviour which sees higher rates of death and injury from suicide, accidents and crime. So there are 'risk factors' and 'protective factors' that impact on the health of men and women (Brown and Harris, 1978). For example, research has suggested that women have stronger social networks than men and can, more easily, rely on contact with close friends and relatives in times of crisis and stress. Marriage may provide a major source of social support, but in a differential way for men and women and across societies. In terms of social support, marriage may be good for men but less so for women. Men tend to rely more on their wives for social support and a confiding relationship, with divorced and widowed men reporting particularly poor health (Payne, 2006).

Activity

Make a list of risks and protective factors that may impact differently on men and women.

What examples of social and cultural change may impact on the health of women.

What do you understand by 'social support' and how might it differ in the lives of men and women?

In the domestic setting of the home there may be disputes about power and the control and management of resources. Pahl showed in a number of studies in the 1990s that in households where men managed and controlled money there were serious consequences for women and children in terms of access to money to spend on food, leisure, clothing, etc. (Pahl, 1990). Her research showed that women and children were most disadvantaged when men controlled and managed household income. In the poorest households, where women had control of money, more was spent on children and on food. In households with male control and management, more was spent on alcohol and male leisure pursuits. Where women's life expectancy is lower than men's it is usually associated with much lower social and economic status. Arber and Thomas (2001) provide a thorough review of the gender inequalities in mortality across different countries. They cite research which shows that excess female mortality is found in countries where women's social status is very low. They write: 'Women's lack of power and influence in the home, and lack of access to valued resources of food, opportunities for leisure, income, may have adverse health consequences' (Arber and Thomas, 2001: 61). International studies show that where women's life expectancy is on a par with men's they are also more likely to be involved in politics, the labour market, and enjoy generally higher levels of economic independence. The national and international variations in morbidity and mortality rates between men and women are a powerful insight into the importance of 'social context' on heath. Despite obvious biological differences, the impact of structural and cultural factors is critical in explaining women's health and the variations between men and women.

Gender and 'emotion work'

In most countries the majority of providers of health and social care are women. This is not an accident but reflects deeply held beliefs and prejudices about the nature of men's and women's personalities, and the most appropriate work for each of them to do. Traditionally, caring roles have been seen as an extension of the 'natural' roles of women. It is they who have usually had major responsibility for the care of children, old people and the sick. Such beliefs are being challenged with the advent of greater equality between men and women.

An obvious example is the changing pattern of paid work in the UK and other countries (Gallie et al., 2001). For example, not only are there many more women in paid work, but they are no longer confined only to 'women's jobs'. More men are entering nursing and the majority of medical students in the UK are now women. Health and social care involves a great deal of what has come to be called 'emotional' labour. The term was coined by Hochschild in her study of the working lives of American flight attendants (Hochschild, 1983). They were required not just to show people to their seats, instruct passengers in safety procedures and serve food and drink. A key part of the job is dealing with the anxieties of passengers while portraying a smiling and confident exterior. They were required to manage their emotions in order to display something they did not necessarily feel.

Social scientists have pointed out that women undertake the bulk of emotional labour in families. Examples of such 'emotion work' include planning household routines, patching up quarrels, arranging family events, remembering birthdays and special occasions, negotiating conflicts, etc. In other words, the domestic work undertaken by women does not just entail physical labour such as housework, but also includes emotional labour. It is obvious that the concept of 'emotional labour' has a great deal of usefulness in understanding the work of provision of health and social care professionals. The delivery of care is not a mechanical process. It involves dealing with people's bodies and their feelings. This may elicit a range of emotions from pity to disgust, fear and sadness. All these emotions must be managed in the encounters between patients, clients and carers.

Activity

If you share your household with others, think of examples of emotional labour being carried out and by whom.

When did you last carry out 'emotion work'?

Are there changes occurring in the amount or type of 'emotion work' being done by men?

Think of examples of how it may be more acceptable for men to display emotion.

From acute to chronic illness

A striking feature of health patterns in rich countries is growing life expectancy for all groups. With this comes the inevitable rise of chronic as opposed to acute illness. Acute illness typically has rapid onset, a fairly predictable course and a clear resolution (death or cure!). Chronic illness on the other hand is more likely to have a slow and insidious onset, sometimes surrounded by uncertainty about diagnosis, prognosis and outcome. The role of professionals is more likely to be about ameliorating the condition and helping to manage its effects. The rise of chronic illness and disability is the dominant characteristic of health care in all industrialised countries. It is obvious that getting a diagnosis of diabetes as opposed to sustaining a leg fracture will have far greater consequences for the person, the professionals who treat them and those who care for them. For the person, a chronic condition might involve a profound and difficult period of adjustment to their new selves. A serious chronic illness involves 'biographical disruption' as many of the expectations people have of their lives and their futures, what they can do in terms of jobs, independence, etc., may have to be rethought and renegotiated. Chronic illness can introduce uncertainty and unpredictability which makes planning all aspects of daily life much more difficult. Chronic and disabling illness may necessitate, therefore, a deep reassessment of oneself as a person (Bury, 1982). In learning to live with a chronic illness it may also be necessary for the sick person to develop a degree of expertise in handling both the illness and the drug treatments. It sometimes comes as a shock to people when they realise that early expectations of medical control over their condition must give way to a recognition that some control of drug balancing lies in their hands (Allott and Robb, 1998).

One of the consequences of this shift from acute to chronic illness is on relationships between professionals and those they care for. There is a strong possibility that people with chronic conditions become so familiar with their own condition through their daily lived experiences that the traditional model of the passive patient is no longer appropriate. In addition, the promotional activities of self-help groups and/or accessing information on the Internet means that many more chronically sick people become expert in their own conditions. If a condition is relatively rare, and professionals encounter it infrequently, it is even more likely that the patient will know more about prognosis and newly emerging treatments than the professionals he or she encounters. This has been acknowledged in the NHS by the 'expert patient' initiative. The changing power balances between professionals and patients/clients means there is potential for much more conflict as the question of 'who knows best?' comes to the fore.

One writer expresses the challenges of chronic illness thus:

> Chronic illness poses more social, interactional, and existential problems than acute illness because it lasts. However, preconceptions of acute illness permeate ideas about chronic illness and pervade institutional practices for handling it. Through analyzing the experience of chronic illness, we learn what chronically ill people's actions mean, when and how they come into conflict with practitioners, and what it means to face loss and reconstruction of self. (Charmaz, 1999: 277)

This author reminds us that the pain, distress and adverse effects of medical procedures cause suffering, but if we concentrate only on physical discomfort we ignore the broader suffering experienced by people who must come to terms with the *loss of self* felt by many persons with chronic illness. In other words, a narrowly medicalised view of suffering might overlook the challenge of coming to terms with a changed self in the context of a society which makes things more difficult than they need be. The disabling effects of wider social expectations are spelt out very clearly by Scambler:

> The lives of the chronically ill are sometimes more restricted than they need to be. The world is set up for the healthy and the able, a fact the ill and disabled usually do not question. Hence, they judge themselves and who and what they should be by yardsticks applied to the healthy and able. In that way, they contribute to the restrictiveness of their own lives. (2003: 166)

In a society which is organised around the healthy and the young, being chronically ill can be a dispiriting experience not just because of the physical limitations caused by the illness. Social attitudes add to the negative experience of chronic illness because, 'experiences of being discredited, embarrassed, ignored and otherwise devalued also contribute to the growing isolation of ill individuals and to their subsequent reappraisals of self' (Scambler, 2003: 169).

Sociologists have also pointed out that we live in an era when the physical appearance of the body has assumed greater significance than ever before for our sense of identity: 'Contemporary society's emphasis on the body makes it a location where much of selfhood is grounded. This emphasis makes it difficult for individuals to dissociate identity from corporeal experience and physical appearance, even when that appearance is flawed' (Gimlin, 2002: 72). If our sense of self and identity is more and more tied up with bodily appearance, it is obvious that physical decline, disability and visible deviations from the 'perfect body' will impact on how we see ourselves and others see us. In western culture conditions which impact on the physicality of the body can lead to negative self-image. This is not invariably the case but there are factors which make it more likely: negative reactions from the outside world, lack of control of bodily functions – we live in a culture which places great emphasis and value on bodily control, or if there is a fear of social or sexual rejection.

Seeking help – the problem of stigma

Decisions to seek help or treatment for particular conditions are not always straightforward. These decisions will be made in the context of quite complex calculations that we all make about the likely costs and benefits of making an appointment to see a doctor or other professional. Among the calculations people are likely to engage in are to weigh up the perceived level of severity of the condition, an assessment of risk and culpability and to what extent there is access to informal care. The visibility of the condition, the extent to which symptoms are 'normalised' and the likelihood of its impinging on functional capacity are also important factors in decisions to seek help. The level of social disapproval of a condition, and the fear of stigma, is one reason why some diseases may be under-reported.

Goffman drew attention to the fact that certain human conditions carry with them the danger of stigma. A stigma originally meant a mark or a scar made with a branding iron that marked out a criminal or a slave. This was a clear sign of outsider or deviant status, visible and unambiguous. Nowadays the term is used more widely to describe any condition or status which marks off a person as 'discredited' in some way. Goffman has shown how these forms of deviance pose particular problems for the sufferer. Because certain conditions, such as mental illness, have been seen as deviant and shameful, it is widely regarded as a stigmatised condition. Some diseases such as HIV/AIDS, leprosy, epilepsy or syphilis are surrounded with vague feelings of disgust or embarrassment and the sufferer has to endure the added problem of a sense of shame or guilt.

Erving Goffman 1922–82

American sociologist and author of *Asylums* in which he describes the process of institutionalisation as a response by patients to the bureaucratic structures imposed on them in total institutions such as mental hospitals, prisons and concentration camps. In 1963 he published *Stigma: Notes on the Management of Spoiled Identity,* which outlines his ideas about the management of stigma. Goffman claims that interpersonal encounters involve performance – hence his use of the term dramaturgical.

The experience of stigma can pose severe barriers to normal social interaction. It can lead to isolation of the individuals, discrimination against them and interrupt the extent and nature of their everyday relationships. Stigmatised individuals experience particular problems in their relations with 'normals'. Victims of stigmatised conditions have suffered abuse, isolation and ridicule. Even if there is no evidence of discrimination, people who are 'discredited', to use Goffman's phrase, will try to manage situations which are made tense or awkward because of their conditions. They have the added difficulty of coping with the reactions of others, in addition to managing their own condition. Public reactions to different diseases will vary in terms of their visibility, obtrusiveness and prevailing attitudes. Of course not all conditions are stigmatised, or those that may be are not stigmatised equally. The onset of chronic arthritis in late middle age is unlikely to lead to the imputation of negative characteristics. Public reactions to different diseases will vary in terms of their visibility, obtrusiveness and prevailing attitudes.

Activity

List three conditions which elicit social disapproval and/or shame and embarrassment.

How might the stigma of a condition be combated?

What are the consequences for the patient/client of suffering from a stigmatised condition?

Think of a condition in which the level of stigma has been reduced in recent times. How has this been achieved?

Even something as common and apparently without stigma as blindness can be seen as a form of deviance. In a classic American study Scott (1969) discovered that the organised socialisation of the blind by medical and welfare agencies was so strong that even some who could see a little came to regard themselves as dependent and adopted the blind role. In his description of cultural stereotyping in the United States, blindness was seen as something that involved docility, helplessness, melancholy and gravity of inner thought. However far-fetched or misleading such stereotyping may be, blind people cannot ignore these beliefs in their interaction with others. How did blind people adapt to such cultural stereotyping in the Scott study? There were a range of reactions from concurring with the dominant view of blindness through to active resistance. Scott also showed how professional interpretations of blindness, and the ways that health and social care workers dealt with blind people, differed across the three countries in which he conducted field work. In the United States the basic goal of the caring professionals was to bring about a therapeutic resolution of the anger of the blind through counselling therapies. The key assumption was the need for the blind to confront and deal with the 'feelings' associated with the loss of their former sighted self. In the UK, at the time of this study there was little effort aimed at therapeutic adjustment. Instead there was an unrelenting cheerfulness in which the professionals saw themselves as combating the melancholy and depression of the blind by always trying to 'keep up their spirits'. In contrast, in Sweden, sight loss was seen as a technical handicap to be addressed by new techniques and aids to daily living. Instead of dealing with the person, effort was directed at changing the external physical environment and training the person with new coping skills. Indeed this approach characterises much of the Scandinavian approach to disability and handicap.

The value of the Scott study is that it shows how varied the responses to a 'deviant' condition can be. Reactions ranged from those who stubbornly resisted the beliefs of health and welfare professionals, through to those who completely accepted their dependent status. Some blind people absorbed or internalised the dominant definitions of the wider society. If professionals and carers, charity workers and friends and family tended to believe that blind people are dependent then that is what they became. Others were able to insulate part of their self-concept from these views and others were able to adopt deliberately a façade of compliance for reasons of expediency. The 'resisters' challenged the stereotyping but this required considerable reserves of power as one of the consequences of rejecting the allotted role is the charge of ingratitude or even bitterness. In the campaigns over disability rights there have certainly been examples of such reactions.

Future challenges and relations between clients and professionals

The term 'professional' has a long and confusing history. It can simply mean the opposite of amateur – as in sports or music. More often it has come to mean work that differs in some important ways from 'just doing a job'. It is also used in an evaluative or judgemental way – to comment negatively or positively on someone's actions or even as a way of commenting on how people dress or speak. This use of 'professional' is not very helpful. It seems best to stick with a definition that stresses 'expertise' and the extent to which people enjoy a degree of freedom in their work, and are able to control the work of others. At one extreme a production line worker or someone responding to enquiries in a call centre enjoys very little autonomy. What they do and say will be the result of careful training, there will be close monitoring and there is almost no scope for individual decision making. At the other end of the spectrum are jobs which enjoy a high level of choice and discretion. Typically medicine has enjoyed high status as a profession and historically doctors as an organised professional group have enjoyed high levels of self-regulation, control over their education and training and control over the work of others.

Activity

Give two examples of occupations that are regarded as 'professions'. Why do they enjoy social prestige?

Give an example of an occupation that is or has been trying to 'professionalise'. What did this involve?

How is it possible to reconcile professional expertise with the wish to involve people in decisions about their care?

Health and social care systems in all rich countries are confronted by a growing 'consumer culture' which has the unintentional effect of eroding traditional deferential approaches to professionals. A generation that endured deprivation and war may be less demanding than a generation brought up during periods of growing affluence and choice. Changing expectations from lay people mean that the scope for tension in the relationship between carers and cared is bound to grow. Certainly doctors have reported much higher levels of dissatisfaction and more conflict in the doctor/patient relationship than in the past. Recent data from the ONS, for example, showed that although around 70 per cent of people were very or quite satisfied with their local NHS doctors or GPs, levels of satisfaction have declined since earlier periods when they were usually around 90 per cent.

Linked to satisfaction is the apparent decline of trust in professionals. A prominent British sociologist has argued that we live in a period in which traditional institutions and authority figures have been undermined (Giddens, 1991). Changes in the status order, raised levels of public education and easier access to information via the Internet mean that many lay people are better equipped than in the past to challenge professional knowledge. As a consequence all professional groups feel the pressure of public scepticism, with their views being treated with much less respect than formerly. There are consequences that flow from this – professionals in health and social care cannot treat their clients and patients as supplicants with the expectation of gratitude. The language of rights and entitlements means that the delivery of care is more likely to be negotiated, and the existence of pressure groups covering every condition and illness gives patients/clients access to information and advice which they can utilise in a power struggle with professional carers. At a time when there is greater scepticism about professionals, and less trust in them, there are also important developments in the training and education of staff to enable them to become more 'professional'. The growth of qualifications such as Foundation Degrees for Health and Social Care professionals, which aim to improve the professional practice of health and social care workers, is part of this process.

How health and social care is funded, organised and delivered in the future is a matter of intense controversy. There will certainly be a very public debate about the relative balance of public and private provision. This underlines a point made at the opening of this chapter that economic, social, ideological and political themes cannot be avoided in future arguments about the funding, organisation and delivery of health and social care. The whole policy area of health and social care is much more contested than in the past. Arguments over NHS and social services rationing are likely to rise up the policy agenda. In the case of the NHS, the President of the Royal College of Surgeons has said that he no longer believes a tax-funded NHS, free at the point of delivery, is sustainable and that it should be abandoned in favour of a social insurance model. According to one newspaper report, 'Many doctors will be surprised and disappointed by his stance, but many also see the need for an intelligent debate about what should be affordable within the NHS' (*Observer*, 14 August 2005). Although the NHS enjoys high levels of public support, and political parties are reluctant to question the funding of health care from taxation, there are voices, particularly on the political right, who note the rising demand for health and social care in the UK and claim that it is unlikely that taxation can continue to be the main basis for funding such services. Research has also shown that people have very high expectations of health and social care services. A poll for the Institute for Public Policy Research found a third believed that the NHS should provide 'all drugs and treatments, no matter what the cost' (*Sunday Telegraph*, 3 September 2006). If state services become more difficult to secure, the burden may well fall more squarely on families, and that usually means women.

The study of the social context of health and social care in coming years will involve recognition of the tensions between differing trends in society. On the one hand we have a growing dependent population as people live longer and more people live alone. There is also evidence of people wanting and expecting more from the health and social care sector as well as being discriminating consumers exercising choice. Professionals in the health and social care sector may be keen to 'empower' the people they care for, and this, along with the rise of the expert patient, challenges deeply held notions of professional superiority. Workers in health and social care face a number of critical challenges over coming decades: How much information to share with those they care for and their families? How can 'clients' become involved in their care? What is the appropriate balance between professional and lay knowledge in decisions about therapy? How might rationing and disputes about priorities affect relations between different professionals? There is no simple answer to any of these dilemmas. What is apparent is that the social trends that affect the demand for health and social care – an ageing population, the rise of disability and chronic illness, smaller families, geographic and social mobility – are likely to continue. This occurs at a time when fewer women are prepared to take on uncomplaining the caring role of the past. Add to this a vigorous consumerism in which we are encouraged to see public services as part of our human rights, and it is clear that the social relations of health and social care can only become more controversial and more contested.

SUMMARY

Health and social care consumes a large and growing proportion of state resources, whether in health spending, social services or on benefits and pensions. Although the state is the main provider in the UK, we can distinguish between care provided by the state, the voluntary sector, the private sector and by lay people (families, friends and neighbours). This is usually referred to as the 'mixed economy' of care. When such large numbers of people (and resources) are

(Continued)

(Continued)

deployed, it is inevitable that decisions about health and social care will involve debates about values, priorities and choices and these are inevitably political. It is also important to differentiate between paid and unpaid care and clarify the different meanings of care. It encompasses a wide variety of relationships and emotions and includes notions of duty, obligation, love, as well as paid care.

Critics of medicine have claimed that the historical benefits of medical interventions have been exaggerated. Some also point out that many treatments and procedures have not been shown to be beneficial. The concept of 'medicalisation' was advanced to draw attention to the extension of medical power and the broadening of the scope of medical interventions in our lives. Critics claim that the medical profession has extended its power and control in societies by claiming jurisdiction over wider areas of life and, in the absence of countervailing sources of moral authority, become the arbiters of how we should live and die. Another facet of the medicalisation argument concentrates on the ever-rising demand for treatments, therapies and drugs to assuage the ills of modern living. There is ample evidence of escalating demand from the public for more consultations, more therapies – conventional, 'alternative' and 'over-the-counter' – as well as more prescriptions. Some critics see this as evidence of socio-cultural trends towards an *individualisation* of problems that have their roots in social and cultural changes. This rising demand for health intervention may be unrelated to any improvements in life expectancy of quality of life but may tell us something about the ways in which, at a societal level, we approach the problems of human living.

Good health and a long life are not distributed equally through societies. Patterns of morbidity and mortality reveal the impact of social class, gender and ethnicity. Inequalities of health are not fixed but fluctuate according to social factors. Although there is real debate about the causes of these inequalities, most explanations come down in favour of either 'structural' or 'cultural' factors or some mix of the two. Rapid social and cultural change impacts on health. Many of the things that impact upon health status are beyond the influence of health services, health professionals or health managers. Deeply rooted gender differences are also seen when we examine 'emotional labour' and the realisation that a great deal of 'emotion work' is done by women in families – and this has obvious relevance for the delivery of health and social care.

Most formal and informal health care in the UK is concerned with managing chronic illness and disability. Because chronic illness is of long-term duration, medical intervention is often about ameliorating symptoms and managing the condition. The consequences of chronic illness can be huge for individuals and their self-identity. It also impacts hugely on their families and friends, and for those who care for them. It has the potential to destabilise traditional relationships between professionals and those they care for, and it calls into question the very basis of 'expert knowledge'. Chronic illness carries with it the threat of stigma. The Greek word *stigma* meant originally a mark or brand burned onto a body to mark a person as a slave. Since then it has come to mean anything that is seen as discreditable about a person. Social and cultural beliefs about particular conditions may impact upon help-seeking behaviour and certain diseases (such as HIV/AIDS) and other conditions (such as mental illnesses) carry with them a degree of shame and/or embarrassment. Professionals need to be aware both of the wider social and cultural understandings about diseases as well as their own beliefs when dealing with patients and clients.

Health and social care professionals face a number of challenges and dilemmas in the early years of the twenty-first century. Important social and cultural changes are occurring that have the potential to transform the relationships between health and social care professionals and those they care for. The rise of a discourse of 'empowerment', human rights and the championing of the 'expert patient' confront professionals with difficult challenges. These ideas challenge traditional notions of professional power and expertise. This could lead to more conflict in the relationship between professionals and those they care for, especially in the context of rising expectations, the rationing of services and a culture of entitlement and 'consumerism'.

Review questions   ?

- What do we mean by the 'mixed economy'?
- Why do health inequalities exist and how might they influence health and social care practice?
- How is the shift from an emphasis on dealing with acute illness to responding to chronic illness affecting health and social care practice?
- Why do health and social care students need an understanding of the concept of medicalisation?
- How might an understanding of stigma help us improve practice?

Further reading

Albrecht, G.L., Fitzpatrick, R. and Scrimshaw, S.C. (eds) (2000) *The Handbook of Social Studies in Health and Medicine.* London: Sage. This is a comprehensive collection covering the main areas of the social context of health and social care with each chapter written by an expert summarising research in areas such as disability, gender, patient satisfaction, medical authority, etc.

Allott, M. and Robb, M. (eds) (1988) *Understanding Health and Social Care: An Introductory Reader.* London: Sage. An interesting and relevant selection of papers covering a wide range of issues in health and social care.

Baggott. R. (2004) *Health and Health Care in Britain*, 3rd edn. Basingstoke: Palgrave Macmillan. This is a comprehensive and readable account of health care in the UK. It has solid, well-written chapters on the development of services and policy dilemmas in health, but with useful summaries of recent policies on community care and patient involvement.

Klein, R. (2002) *The New Politics of the NHS*, 4th edn. London: Prentice Hall. A classic study of the politics of the NHS since its creation. It is invaluable because it puts into historical context much of the hype around the 'crisis' of the NHS.

Nettleton, S. (2006) *The Sociology of Health and Illness,* 2nd edn. Cambridge: Polity Press. Highly regarded, clearly written sociology textbook in an up-to-date second edition that covers many issues of relevance to health and social care including social inequalities, lay–professional interactions and chronic illness.

Payne, S. (2006) *The Health of Men and Women.* Cambridge: Polity Press. A more advanced summary of the theories and evidence about the differences and similarities in the health of men and women. The book discusses a range of health-related behaviours such as diet, exercise, alcohol, smoking and drug use.

5 | VALUES IN PRACTICE

Steven Parker

SUMMARY CHAPTER CONTENTS

- Defining values
- Understanding values, moral principles and ethics
- Ethical principles in health and social care
- Empowerment
- A practice model for working with values

Learning objectives

By the end of this chapter, you should be able to:

■ Engage with the debate around the moral principles and values that underpin good practice in health and social care.

■ Understand the idea of empowering practice.

■ Reflect on what it means to be a morally active practitioner.

■ Uphold the fundamental rights of people who use care services.

■ Recognise how practitioners have to work with conflicting values, opinions, beliefs and attributes, and the resulting ethical issues which influence practice.

Introduction

As practitioners we intervene in people's lives. We need to know that our interventions do no harm and that we are doing the 'right' thing; our practice thus becomes a moral activity.

Our practice becomes guided by values (Beckett and Maynard, 2005). Dawson and Butler (2003) make this clear when they say that to be morally active is 'to act on the basis of internal values' rather than solely rely on externally imposed codes of conduct.

Tensions and conflicts may exist between values resulting in ethical dilemmas and problems (Banks, 2006; Eby, 2000b). Importantly this chapter will enable you to examine how as practitioners you may have to work with conflicting values, opinions, beliefs and attributes, and the resulting ethical issues and develop a value-based framework to reflect upon your practice.

By making links between a range of issues this chapter should equip you with a sound understanding of the moral principles that underpin practice and you will have a clear understanding of empowering practice as a central moral principle. Students will be in a position of being morally active practitioners who believe in the fundamental rights of people who use care services.

Defining values

The idea that practitioners in health and social care have a set of values that they should work to permeates professional practice. Dawson and Butler (2003) suggest that social care workers need to be aware of the importance of values and so have an ethical framework to do their job. Banks (2000) argues that a practitioner would need 'to be aware of the societal and professional values underlying her work and her own values' (2000: 64).

Thompson (1995) suggests that values are not just applicable to the social work profession but broadly applicable to the helping professions.

For Eby (2000b: 118) values are 'beliefs, ideas, and assumptions that individuals and groups hold about themselves and the society they live in'. Our personal set of values guide our daily lives. There is a complex interaction between our values and the culture and norms of society and the community in which we belong. Values both inform and are informed by our surroundings.

Martin and Henderson (2001: 57) tell us that 'values are deep seated beliefs about what is right or wrong'. It is this central belief of what is right and wrong, that guides our daily life and professional action.

The decisions we make when intervening in someone else's life are informed by our moral position and that makes any intervention in someone else's life a moral activity. So as practitioners we need to practise in a way that is morally and ethically right and for Husband (1995) this means we need to be morally active practitioners.

Davies (1981) pointed out over 25 years ago that social (care) workers are in a position of power and authority. His message continues to be applicable today: that practitioners need to be aware of their power in relation to people who use social and health care services. As they intervene in people's lives, practitioners need to be aware of their position in the web of power, which surrounds people who use services.

Our value base needs to take into account this inferred authority as we make ethical decisions about and intervene in the lives of people who use health and social care services.

Martin and Henderson (2001) point out that values are held at different levels. Values are held and shared by society at large, by organisations, by groups or teams of people, or at an individual level. They suggest that these values interact and influence each other.

Understanding values, moral principles and ethics

Dawson and Butler (2003) equate the terms ethical and moral, so to be morally active is to act ethically. To think and act ethically and morally right requires a set of values (Dawson and Butler, 2003) and so practitioners need to develop an ethical perspective to their work.

Activity: Values and moral principles

What do you consider to be the principles that guide your life?
What do you believe to be right and wrong?

Practitioners in health and social care hold sets of values or ethical principles that can be understood in terms of moral philosophy. Raphael (1994) defines moral philosophy as exploring ideas of right and wrong, good and bad, what should and should not be done. This moral philosophy of practice is used to guide practice, it cannot tell practitioners what to do, but it can enable practitioners to explore the dilemmas of practice decisions. By exploring the different ethical approaches practitioners can reflect on ethical dilemmas they encounter and clarify the issues that are created when intervening in people's lives. The choice of what decision to make remains with you, the health and social care practitioner.

To understand and reflect on the ethical issues in practice to enable practitioners to be morally active it is useful to explore some general approaches to understanding the area of moral principles and ethics that have developed over time. The principles that exist within the domain of moral philosophy can act as a framework to examine our own values and the professional ethical principles that have come to influence our practice.

Utilitarian principles

The basic premise of utilitarianism is that the right action is that which produces the greatest balance of good over harm. As Raphael (1994) points out, the right action is the action that produces most happiness. So actions are right if they result in good and remove or prevent what is bad. The principle of utilitarianism has been discussed and debated over the past 150 years or so and has resulted in a range of variations.

Traditional utilitarianism according to Raphael (1994) attempts to simplify the concept to the idea that 'things are valued for the sake of pleasure, either the pleasure they themselves contain or the pleasure they are likely to produce'.

Other notions of utility such as hedonistic utilitarianism suggest that the pursuit of pleasure alone is to be regarded as good. Ideal utilitarianism would say that other things could be regarded as good other than pleasure, such as love, virtue, knowledge, and beauty.

The consequences of actions can be linked to utilitarian principles in that the morality of an action can be determined by whether or not its consequences are seen as good (Beckett and Maynard, 2005). This can be broken down into act and rule utilitarianism. Act utilitarianism is where the morality of a person's actions are judged by their consequences and whether they result in the greatest amount of good. Rule utilitarianism is where the rules which cover actions can be judged as contributing to the greatest good (Beckett and Maynard, 2005).

The principles inherent within utilitarianism seem to offer an overarching framework for action: that what we do in our practice should produce the greatest amount of good and happiness for the people we work with. For Banks (2000), though, the principles of utility 'tells us nothing about whose good' we should be promoting. In the delivery of health and social care services should we be promoting what people who use the service regard as being good, to promote happiness and utility as defined by the people who access the services they need? Or should we be promoting what others view as good, such as society, or what we as practitioners would call 'in someones' best interest'?

Banks (2000) suggests that utilitarian principles have not been well developed in social care work, as they do not seem to account for the central personal relationship inherent in social care work practice.

Kantian principles: respect for the person and individualism

Raphael (1994) believes that Kantian principles are more satisfying in suggesting a single moral framework, other than when it comes to conflicts between rules. For Raphael, Kantian principles are about three things:

- When making a moral decision we should treat everyone in the same way.
- We should treat people as always having 'ends' and not merely as 'means'. By this Kant is saying that we should regard people as having a purpose, a purpose made up of 'desires' and 'choices' and an ability to make decisions. It is a moral duty to enable people to carry out their own decisions. It then becomes morally wrong to dominate other people, to exert power over others, to treat them as a 'means'. It also becomes morally wrong to fail to help where help is needed.
- We should be collectively making decisions. We should accept that other people are competent, suggesting a concept of equality. Thus, 'every human being equally has the power to make choices and decisions'.

For Kant there is recognition that everyone has unconditional worth and the power to make decisions and the moral capacity to determine their own moral destiny. It would also seem that we all have a moral duty to enable this to happen.

Banks (2000) suggests that neither Kantian nor utilitarian principles can provide a single principle for determining the right action. Instead she notes that authors on professional ethics draw upon both when thinking about moral issues.

Virtue ethics

Recently the idea of virtue ethics has become important in health and social care.

Kantian and utilitarian approaches for understanding moral decision making have been criticised for being directive and used to predict courses of action.

Acting within a Kantian framework of obligation one may be accused of simply doing one's duty rather than because one wanted to do the right thing. To be a virtuous person is to do the right thing because you want to do the right thing. It is not simply because it is your duty to do the right thing.

Within a utilitarian framework you may determine your actions after considering the consequences of your action. Your intervention could be based on a realisation that the result will not be of 'good' or most benefit.

As an alternative approach, being virtuous is based on your moral character and capacity. You are doing the right thing because you believe in the right thing. It is, as Beauchamp and Childress (2001) say, about doing the right thing from 'the right state of mind'. The idea of being a virtuous person is a socially valued human characteristic.

McBeath and Webb (2002) point out that virtues are 'acquired inner qualities' that when applied 'contribute to the realisation of the good life'. So the idea of having a virtue is a concept that makes the person good. Being virtuous could be synonymous with being a morally good person, of having a moral character.

Beauchamp and Childress (2001) suggest that it becomes impossible to identify and assess a range of virtues presumably because the traits of character that can be regarded as being a virtue could be endless. Despite this difficulty they do identify 'central virtues' of:

- Compassion: being an active regard for another person's welfare and an ability to have empathy.
- Discernment: being about being able to make decisions with sensitive insight.
- Trustworthiness: concerned with being able to be relied upon, of having the moral character and competence that other people can rely upon.
- Integrity: concerned with being a morally reliable person and able to stand up for the principles that one believes in.
- Conscientiousness: being about doing the right thing because it is right and having given some thought to what may be the right action.

Virtues in social care have been explored by McBeath and Webb (2002) who identify social (care) workers as being able to apply the virtues of:

- Justice
- Reflection
- Perception
- Judgement
- Bravery
- Prudence
- Liberality
- Temperance.

For McBeath and Webb (2002) social (care) workers require these virtues to make judgements based on the workers' perception and judgement and not on an automated response based on organisational requirements. Virtuous social care workers are able to reflect on their action and to strive to do the right thing.

Radical agenda

Shardlow (2002) comments that a new set of values have emerged over the past 20 years, which are concerned with challenging discrimination and oppression and the promotion of equality (Thompson, 2003). The radical approach to values attempts to address issues of power and oppression.

Such values have been differentiated from traditional values, which seem to focus on the individual relationship between the professional practitioner and the person requiring a service. Such traditional values could be said to reflect an individualisation of supporting or even empowering people. The radical agenda, as Banks (2000) points out, acknowledges the role of social (care) workers as agents of control on behalf of an oppressive system. The need for social work as a profession to acknowledge the need to reflect an anti-oppressive agenda was incorporated into professional values.

In working in a way that challenges structural oppression, social care workers need to recognise that the 'very rules and structures within which society operates reflect basic inequalities in power' (Banks, 2000: 59). This can be a challenging concept for social and health care workers.

Banks (2000) also points out that radical approaches focus on the structures that cause problems such as poverty, poor housing, patriarchy or racism. Interventions in people's lives become part of a wider agenda of enabling people to recognise that they are an oppressed group and so develop their ability to 'work collectively for social change'. Traditional values are seen as a system of rules and principles that maintain the oppression of people because they reflect the interests of the powerful dominant groups in society. Radical values then reflect the idea that social (care) workers should enable people to exercise more choice, be part of the decision-making process, and be in control.

Radical values are reflected in the ideas of anti-discriminatory practice (Thompson, 2006) and the promotion of equality (Thompson, 2003). Thompson (2001, 2003) believes that an essential principle of practice is that good practice must be anti-discriminatory practice. Anti-discriminatory and anti-oppressive practices are seen as essential values to be upheld.

Values in health and social care tend to be dominated by Kantian principles of respecting the person, and utilitarian principles relating to the promotion of the wider good. Practitioners are also taking on board the radical agenda and acknowledge their role as virtuous people.

Ethical principles in health and social care

Health and social care practitioners have a history of ethical guidance and principles which enable them to develop what Beauchamp and Childress (2001) regard as a professional morality. A profession shares this morality as it is common amongst practitioners who acknowledge their moral responsibilities.

In the area of health, Beauchamp and Childress (2001) outline a framework of moral principles. They regard their set of moral principles as 'guidelines for professional ethics', namely:

- Respect for autonomy
- Nonmaleficence
- Beneficence
- Justice.

In social (care) work Banks (2000) believes that it is possible to determine four principles:

- Respect for and promotion of individual rights to self-determination
- Promotion of welfare or well-being
- Equality
- Distributive justice.

The principles above have similarities and differences and are relevant to the practice of health and social care workers.

Respect for autonomy: the promotion of individual rights to self-determination

By autonomy at a personal level Beauchamp and Childress (2001) mean the freedom to act as people wish. An autonomous person is able to choose and is not controlled by others. Ideas around autonomy link to notions of freedom and liberty so that individuals are free from controlling influences. For Beauchamp and Childress (2001), being autonomous means that people have a right to 'hold views', 'choose, and act on their own beliefs'.

Banks' principle of self-determination is similar. She regards self-determination in two ways: as allowing people to do what they choose, and creating the conditions which enable people to become more self-determining. So, as practitioners this means that we need to practise in a way that promotes and enables people to be autonomous. It also means that our practice should actively enable people to be autonomous.

Both authors point out that it is important to determine a person's capacity to be self-determining. For Banks this will be limited by judgements of the person's competence, the need for protection and the right to participate. She also suggests that being self-determining may not be without its limitations, as in the interests of justice it may not be possible to promote the rights of service users at the expense of others.

This view of autonomy, though, is quantified by Beauchamp and Childress (2001) who believe that the obligation to respect autonomy does not extend to people who cannot act in a sufficiently autonomous manner and therefore cannot be regarded as autonomous. This would include people who, as health and social care practitioners, we would be working with.

Activity: Reflecting on respecting personal autonomy

What do you think would limit personal autonomy?

Should 'incapacity' limit autonomy?

Who defines who is capable or not in having the right to make decisions and choose?

Beauchamp and Childress (2001) also suggest that a person's autonomy is reduced by their capacity to make decisions for themselves. In social and health care, practitioners need to respect the autonomy of individuals to make decisions and choices for themselves. Beauchamp and Childress (2001) limit this autonomy on grounds of mental capacity, suggesting that people with learning difficulties may not be able to be autonomous due to 'limited capacity for intentional action'.

These views of autonomy and self-determination raise a number of issues for practitioners working with people with cognitive impairments. Do such people have the same rights as other people to be autonomous? How much power does a person seen as having cognitive impairment have to determine or make decisions about the service they are involved in? Some of these issues may be answered as we look at a central value of empowerment.

Activity: Shopping

Belinda is a young woman living in the community after spending over 10 years in a long-stay hospital. The staff that work with her have a professional remit to encourage Belinda's independence. This includes learning how to go shopping. For the care workers working with Belinda this means encouraging Belinda to shop at the local supermarket.

Belinda says she does not want to go shopping. She found the experience stressful and uncomfortable.

The organisational response is to help Belinda go shopping by using established learning methods, breaking down the task by a task analysis, teaching the process in small stages and eventually withdrawing, so that Belinda can shop independently.

The justification behind this is that Belinda needs to be independent and it is the role of social care staff to encourage this. It is also an organisational aim of community care.

o   To what extent do you believe that Belinda's views be considered?

o   Should she be forced to go shopping against her will?

o   How far do you think Belinda should determine her own destiny?

o   What are your views concerning independence?

o   To what degree, if any, should incapacity limit autonomy?

Nonmaleficence

For Beauchamp and Childress (2001) the principle of nonmaleficence is an obligation to do no harm. As practitioners we need to know that our actions when we intervene in people's lives do no harm. It is about not implementing any action that may cause harm to anyone.

In some instances society may endorse harming other people by placing them in prison and other forms of punishment.

Principles of not causing harm can be recognised when looked at in terms of causing no pain, or not to kill someone, but how as social care practitioners are we able to determine if our actions and interventions do not cause harm?

Beneficence and the promotion of welfare or well-being

Beneficence and the promotion of welfare is about providing benefit and 'good' to people. This is different from the ideas of nonmaleficence as beneficence is a positive act to help other people, not simply to refrain from harming them.

Beauchamp and Childress (2001) argue that practitioners should contribute to the welfare of people and make a positive contribution to help other people. They see the principles of beneficence as being distinguishable from the virtue of benevolence and being a positive action where intended to benefit another person.

Banks (2000) points out that the promotion of good is open to interpretation. The definition of what is good can be socially and culturally determined. What is a good quality of life? And who determines it? Who determines what is in a person's best interest? The professional or the person who uses the service?

So there is a moral obligation to act for the benefit of other people.

Beneficence and the promotion of welfare are linked to utilitarian principles in the sense that they may involve the balancing of action to determine the action which provides the greatest benefit.

Justice and distributive justice

The moral principle of justice for Beauchamp and Childress (2001) is concerned with inequality in accessing services. Justice can be seen as fair, equitable and appropriate treatment.

Distributive justice is about the fair, equitable and appropriate distribution of all rights and responsibilities in society including civil and political rights. For Banks, distributive justice can be according to certain rules and criteria, which can be selected from people's existing rights, 'desert' and need. This is a fundamental part of social care work that practitioners are involved in and are responsible for the distribution of public resources according to set eligibility criteria and assessment of need.

The principle of justice is about treating people equally and fairly.

Equality

Equality is linked to the principle of justice and can for some be within the concept of justice. For Banks it is about 'the removal of disadvantage' and can be regarded in different ways.

The idea of equal treatment may provide some basic principle that people should not be treated disadvantageously by discrimination and prejudice, but as Bagihole (1997) points out, this does not tackle the complex interaction between the social, political and economic issues surrounding the concept of equality. Equality of opportunity is the 'provision of equality of access to institutions and social positions amongst relevant social groups' (Bagihole, 1997: 32).

For social care workers this may include 'the removal of disadvantage in competition with others, giving people the means to achieve socially desired ends' (Banks, 2000: 39). This would for instance enable the same access to information for people who do not read as people who do read, information about services being made available to people in symbols, for instance.

Enabling equality of access does not tackle issues of equality of condition. Equality of condition is about recognising the material and cultural disadvantages that some groups in society have. So Bagihole (1997) suggests that inequalities of condition can obstruct real equalities of opportunity as people are not starting from the same position.

Equality of result or outcome is a radical approach to equal opportunity which is about applying differing policies and procedures to different social groups in an attempt to remove past discrimination and disadvantage. This becomes the application of preferential treatment to different groups because 'past disadvantages require us to treat people unequally' (Jenks, 1988, quoted in Bagihole, 1997: 33).

For Banks, social (care) workers are involved in the differing forms of promoting equality. She suggests that equality of treatment is easier to achieve, and this also fits in with the moral principle of respecting the person. Equality of opportunity may require policy decisions while equality of result involves practitioners with the radical agenda of tackling oppression and discrimination.

Thompson (2003) regards equality as a complex concept but sees the idea as essentially concerning itself with human rights and that as social care workers an essential component of the work we do is to address inequality and promote social justice.

The idea of having a set of principles to guide practice is not without its problems. How do we know which set of moral principles we should be using at any one particular point in time or in any one situation? Beauchamp and Childress (2001) see moral principles not as separate entities but being used in a combined way. The skill for you as a practitioner is to be able to recognise the moral principles at play, recognise the dilemmas these create, and to act in a way that reflects what you believe to be the right action in the process of being morally active. There is a need to be aware of the competing values and moral principles because, unless we are, it may be easy to favour one over all the others without fully recognising the ethical issues presented in our practice and interventions in people's lives. Dawson and Butler (2003) suggest that principles concerning the autonomy of people tend to be concentrated upon at the expense of the others. As practitioners it is important not simply to advocate autonomy at the expense of other moral considerations.

Competing values, ethical issues and dilemmas

Values themselves are held at different levels. Martin and Henderson (2001) point out that values are held at a societal, organisational, team and individual level and that these different levels interact and influence each other. It will be inevitable that tensions and conflicts may exist between values at the different levels. These tensions will sometimes result in ethical dilemmas and problems for social and health care workers (Banks, 2000; Eby, 2000b).

Societies and cultures across the globe have a diverse range of values, of what is believed to be right or wrong. This diversity is replicated, complicated and transformed in modern industrialised/pluralistic societies where there is no one defining culture and where differing values, codes and rules exist side by side, and become integrated and transformed into new ideas of what is right or wrong. In this sense societal values are not static but transform over time and territory.

The organisational values within health and social care reflect the values of society but also the government of the time. The policy of government will influence the values of the organisations delivering services. The values of health and social care organisations are reflected in their policy statements and community action plans, mission statements and health action plans.

Activity: Societal and organisational values

Go to www.dh.gov.uk and search for 'National and Local Plans'. You can refine your search by looking for services that you are interested in.

o What societal and organisational values are reflected in these national and local standards?
o Do they reflect Kantian principles or utilitarian principles?
o Do the service plans and national standards reflect a service user perspective?
o Do they promote the involvement of people at a radical level?
o Is the government virtuous in its action?

Working in teams is an integral part of health and social care. As a practitioner you may well find yourself as part of a team. A team is a group of people who are working together towards a common aim. The team has a shared task, and in terms of health and social care this shared task will be to provide a service to people who use that service. The team may also have a shared set of values influenced by the professional organisation it works for and the people who use the service.

As health and social care services increasingly work collaboratively and in partnership with other agencies and organisations there may well be differences in professional values appearing. As services move towards integration with differing professional groups coming together, there may well be the formation of new integrated values. There may also be the possibility of a clash of values between different professional groups with differing professional ideologies.

Individual values

We will all hold our individual beliefs of what is right or wrong. Our individual values can be held at a personal level and have developed over time from our own upbringing, socialisation and experiences. It is these values held at a personal level that guide our individual actions. We also hold sets of professional values derived from our professional training and professional ideology. These values are reflected in codes of conduct and reinforced by the profession we belong to. The professional decisions we make will reflect our professional and personal values.

As values are held at these different levels and influence each other there may well be conflicts between values when intervening and making decisions which affect people's lives. All the decisions we make and interventions in people's lives have an ethical dimension. In some instances values may conflict or be in competition with other values. How as a practitioner can you decide which value or moral principle overrides the other?

Eby (1994; 2000b) points out that ethical problems arise when there is a conflict between competing values and principles, and this results in ethical distress or creates an ethical dilemma. Ethical distress is when a barrier prevents a course of action. In such situations the values of the organisation may conflict with your own personal individual values. What you believe is right cannot be enacted because the organisation has other priorities.

An ethical dilemma is when you have a choice to make between moral principles. In one instance there is a choice between equally right courses of action; the decision is which morally right decision to make between the two. The other instance is whatever decision you make will result in a compromise of values or principles. How do you decide?

Ethical dilemmas can occur between competing values at the personal individual level and competing values held at different levels such as the individual and organisational and within teams. As a practitioner you will need to make decisions about what is right or wrong when intervening in someone's life.

To enable health and social care workers to make ethical decisions it is important that practitioners develop the skills of being reflective. As health and social care practitioners it is important to reflect on the ethical decisions we make and be aware of the conflicts and tensions that may occur when making decisions about people. Reflecting and thinking about the ethical dimension of your work and the decisions that you have to make enables you to develop a moral framework for your practice. Your moral framework helps you make the decisions that you need to.

The morally active practitioner

It is important to reflect on your role as a social and health care practitioner, to look at the wider social context of the work you are doing, the moral and ethical base of your work, and your guiding moral and ethical principles.

As we briefly mentioned in Chapter 2, Husband (1995) suggests that we need to be morally active practitioners and act as autonomous moral agents. The morally active practitioner uses internal values rather than externally imposed codes of conduct to guide his or her ethical decision making. The morally active practitioner would therefore recognise professional ethics as external guidelines backed by external pressures of professional bodies.

This is not to say that ethical guidelines are not desirable, but practitioners should not hide behind 'ethical anaesthesia' but keep their responsibility for their own professional practice.

Codes of practice become a method by which professional morality is formalised and codified. Codes often become rules as well as reflecting professional moral obligations and they reinforce the professional values.

Activity: Codes of conduct as moral principles

Instructions

Choose a professional area that is of interest to you and use an Internet search for the relevant code of professional conduct.

For instance:

o For social care work: Go to the General Social Care web site at www.gscc.org.uk and follow the links to the codes of practice. The codes are available as PDF files or as a Word document.

o For social work: Go to The British Association of Social Work web site at www.basw.co.uk and search for codes of ethics.

o For health care (nursing): Go to the Nursing Midwifery Council at www.nmc-uk.org and via 'Popular Links' go to NMC Codes of Conduct.

- View or download the codes of conduct or practice.

- Using the information you have read so far, explore to what extent professional codes of conduct can be regarded as moral principles.

- o Are the codes complete?
- o Does following the codes mean that a practitioner has met his or her moral obligations?
- o What if a practitioner has a conflict with the code?
- o Are practitioners free to operate outside the code and be morally active?
- o What moral and ethical dilemmas are created by conflicting codes?
- o To what extent do you believe that codes of conduct may restrict your ethical decision making or support your ability to be a morally active practitioner?

Empowerment

To aid decision making it is worthwhile to consider empowerment as a central and core value and principle to underpin your practice and develop your understanding of being morally active. The notion of service user empowerment can be seen as a central moral principle and can be used as a basis to reflect upon your practice as a morally active practitioner.

Gillon (1994, quoted in Dawson and Butler, 2003) sees empowerment as the combination of the moral principles of beneficence and the respect for autonomy. It is also concerned with tackling issues of equality and social justice. As we explore empowerment we can see how as a central value it can combine the range of moral principles. Empowerment also embraces the moral principles of Beauchamp and Childress and the ideas of Banks.

A moral principle of empowerment is not incompatible with Kantian principles of respecting people as being able to make choices and decisions about their lives. Nor is it incompatible with doing the greater good, especially if the greater good is about what people want from services to meet their own needs. And a virtuous person would surely not want to be part of the oppression of less powerful people.

Shardlow (2002) sees empowerment of individuals as being part of the radical agenda rather than within the traditional framework of professional values. Yet this seems to have shifted as the principle of empowering people becomes part of the mainstream agenda in health and social care. Rather than being a radical value it has become an accepted moral premise.

The notion of empowering people who use services is central to the government rhetoric in health and social care. The Department of Health sees service user involvement as an essential component of the vision of the future of adult care services as outlined in the Green Paper *Independence Well Being and Choice*.

The Social Care Institute for Excellence also promises to promote service user empowerment and the Commission for Social Care Improvement acknowledges that empowerment is an important issue for service users.

The problem is, as Gomm (1993) has pointed out, 'empowerment' has become something of a buzzword and can mean different things to different people. Shardlow (2002) identifies empowerment as a new value which challenges oppression and suggests that there are different theoretical approaches to empowerment. For Payne (1997), empowerment is about helping people gain power of decisions and actions over their own lives. Adams (2003) defines empowerment as the way people are 'able to take control of their circumstances and achieve their own goals' (2003: 8). Thompson (2003) suggests that it is important that practitioners need to be clear about what it means. We will explore different models of empowering practice in an attempt to clarify its meaning and so enable you to use the ideas as a framework to develop an empowering value base.

Given that health and social care practitioners are in a position of power and work explicitly with people in vulnerable positions, it becomes increasingly important for practitioners to evaluate their own practice and examine their own position of power and potential to develop empowering practice as a moral activity.

Power and empowerment

To understand the concept of empowerment we need to look at the idea of power. What is meant by power and how does it affect the people we work with and how can we use power to benefit the people we work with?

Allen (2000) looks at the different forms that power takes in society. Power can be seen in terms of actions such as coercion, manipulation, domination, constraints, expertise, authority and persuasion. Thompson (2003) sees power as 'the ability to influence and control people, events processes or resources'. There is a positive side to power which enables things to be done, but there is also a flip side in which power can be destructive, exploitatitive, oppressive or abusive. Thompson makes it quite clear that social care workers need to understand issues concerning the idea of power if we are to promote equality as a moral principle and so work in an empowering way.

As a social care practitioner you will find yourself in positions that reflect an amount of power in relation to the people you work with. You may have some influence over decisions which affect the service people will receive, decisions based on the resources that are available to provide the services that people say they need. Your knowledge of which services are available or to offer places you in a position of power in relation to the person requiring your service. Your theoretical understanding of issues and knowledge of research-based evidence place you in a position of power. The organisation you work for may have mandates to provide services as well as statutory duties to intervene in people's lives. As soon as you enter into the life of another person, you are the face and personal representative of a powerful organisation.

It is useful to look at this concept of being in a position of power within a theoretical framework. Allen (2000) and Thompson (2003) both refer to Weberian concepts and the ideas of Foucault to explain power.

In a Weberian sense welfare organisations such as health and social care agencies can be regarded as bureaucratic organisations, with clear hierarchical structures. There are people in definite positions of power. The structure of the organisation resembles a pyramid and this hierarchy legitimises and reinforces people's position and their power in relation to other people. There are lines of accountability and systems such as supervision and the allocation of tasks, roles and responsibilities also maintain everyone's position.

In contrast to this model of power Foucault (in Allen, 2000; Thompson, 2003) sees power as something that is all around us. Rather than being controlled by those above us in the hierarchy, power is seen as a guiding force and we control ourselves due to the practices and systems of society and the organisation which are all interconnected in a complex web. Power is not simply from above but fully encompasses us. Within this complex web of systems and processes we all know our place and we all tend to comply.

Looking at your position and power

Listed in the activities below are some areas to reflect upon that arise from Allen's (2000) discussion of power.

Activity

Have a look at these questions and consider them in relation to your practice experience using a Weberian framework.

As a health or social care worker:

o How do you fit into a hierarchical structure of the agency you work for?
o Where are your lines of accountability?
o How is power exercised through systems of supervision and accountability?
o Who is *in* authority?
o Who is *an* authority?
o What tasks are delegated to you and how is power delegated to you?
o How do rules and procedures govern your practice?
o What discretion do you have in the work you undertake?

- o How does your position of power reflect a hierarchical structure?
- o Who further up the hierarchy knows about your day-to-day practice?
- o Where does your position of power come from when working with service users?

From the ideas of Foucault power has a much more anonymous feel. Consider the following questions in terms of power being a guiding force and people regulating themselves.

- o Why do you comply with the expectations of your role as a health or social care practitioner?
- o How are people who use services forced to accept your position as a health and social care worker?
- o How do people know how to play the role associated with being:

  (a) a member of society;
  (b) a senior member of staff;
  (c) a health and social care practitioner; or
  (d) someone who uses services?

- o How is your practice observed and monitored?
- o How is your practice constantly monitored?
- o In what ways does it feel like your practice is being observed?
- o How does the web of power influence your practice and your relationship with the people you work with?

Models of empowerment in health and social care

A range of differing models of empowerment exist to promote the welfare of people and shift the balance of power from service providers and professionals to people who use services in the promotion of equality.

Normalisation and social role valorisation

The principle of normalisation has been extremely influential in the development of community-based services in the UK since the 1980s. Different strands of the theoretical underpinnings of normalisation developed in Scandinavia, the United States and also in the UK. It is seen as a model of empowerment because it called for people to be able to access everyday services in the community, such as housing, education, employment, transport and recreational facilities.

Normalisation has its roots in the work of Erving Goffman and his concept of stigma. Goffman (1963) states that if a person is seen to be different and be seen as a 'less desired kind' of person by others that person becomes 'tainted'.

The ideas around normalisation are designed to counter stigma so that a person has a valued role and their 'undesired differences are reduced'. The principles underlying this concept have led to the ideas that people should be enabled to live ordinary lives, enjoy the benefits of living in the community and be regarded as part of the community and society with valued roles. Living an ordinary life is seen as a socially valued concept and something that should remove stigma and discrimination. Long-term institutions were closing and it was seen as right that people should live in the community rather than be excluded from the mainstream of society.

Wolfensberger and Tullman (1982) define the principle of normalisation as 'the use of culturally valued means in order to enable, establish and/or maintain valued social roles for people'. Wolfensberger (1998) later elaborated on his concept and renamed his idea social role valorisation. He is very clear that:

> in order for people to be treated well by others, it is very important that they be seen as occupying valued roles ... [and that] ... the greater number of valued roles a person ... occupies, the more likely it is that [they] will be accorded those good things of life. (Wolfensberger, 1998: 58)

He also goes on to suggest that it is a value judgement of the professional as to whether or not a person should be valued by others.

So for Wolfensberger, service provision should be based on the creation and establishment of socially valued roles. If services promoted positive roles for people, the negative consequences of being labelled would diminish. Wolfensberger suggests some very specific examples of how devalued people should be to improve their chances of being socially valued. This includes for example the notion that people should wear appropriate clothing so as to fit in with social situations. Thus people become valued for fitting into the mainstream.

The concept was embraced by social work professionals to improve the lives of people coming out of long-term institutions. Professional practice reflected the need to provide people with opportunities to experience valued social positions and these opportunities would deal with how people were treated as non-valued citizens. The ideas of social role valorisation continue to influence practice and national policy (DoH, 2001).

Despite their influence on services the ideas of normalisation and social role valorisation have been criticised on a number of levels. Scott (1970) suggests that in responding to stigma professionals create their own conception of stigma reflecting the 'social, cultural and economic environments' of which the professional is a part. In this sense normalisation as a response to stigma can be seen as a professional construction of an identity for a person based upon professional expectations of being a person who is stigmatised.

As Brown and Walmsley (1997) point out, service based on these principles may reject the need for services that are designed to meet individual need. The emphasis on normally valued roles and services could be at the expense of meeting specialised need and place the need for change with the individual rather than with the structures of society.

Normalisation also has an emphasis on integration and relationships with people who are regarded as not being stigmatised rather than collective action. The condition responsible for the stigmatisation of an individual is placed with the person rather than the organisation of society and the ideas of what is regarded as positive perpetuated by a dominant ideology.

Normalisation has had a significant impact on empowering service users and has changed the face of service delivery from institutional care to community-based services. This should not be ignored, but as a basis for making value-based decisions and as a model of empowerment it needs to be questioned. People should be valued as people, not for the roles they have. It is a professional model devised and implemented by professionals with little or no input from the people who use services. We need to look at other models of empowerment as moral principles.

Advocacy

Despite the good intentions of service providers and professionals, some people who use services simply do not have their voices heard. A range of issues may be responsible for people's voices not being acknowledged, from a service that is not reciprocal or acknowledging that people have different methods of communication to implicit disempowerment of individuals by others in positions of power. Goodley and Ramcharan (2005) suggest that people's views, aspirations and ambitions are dismissed because of the view that some people have nothing important to say and that because of different cognitive abilities people lack the awareness to say anything of any worth. People's views are dismissed because people do not know what is best for them or it is the professional who is the one who knows the most appropriate course of action.

To enable people's voices to be heard the practice of advocacy has entered into health and social care practice. The central idea of advocacy is defined by Goodley and Ramcharan as that a 'person speaks for themselves or that an advocate speaks for that person as if that person's voice were their own' (2005: 152).

This raises a number of issues about enabling people to speak up for themselves and the position of the advocate. The systems need to be in place which enable people to voice their concerns and opinions concerning their services, about being involved in the decisions that are made about them; people's voices need to be recognised as being valuable and their views taken on board. This approach to advocacy presents challenges to social care workers and organisations as it is a challenge to professional and organisational power. Advocates also need to be able to voice the views of other people without any judgement of that view. To voice another's view as if it was his or her own, an advocate would need to represent that view regardless of his or her own views. The advocate's role is simply to represent the views of someone so that the view is heard and taken seriously.

A number of different models of advocacy (see Table 5.1) have developed over the past 20 years with different characteristics and qualities.

TABLE 5.1   *TYPES OF ADVOCACY*

Types of advocacy	Characteristics	Weaknesses
Citizen advocacy	Unpaid volunteers linked with a person offering one-to-one support	There can be a difficulty in the recruitment and training of volunteers
	Volunteers are trained in advocacy skills and are able to represent the views of the person they are working with	There can be a skills gap in the requirements of being an advocate
	The relationship can be mutual and significant for both the advocate and partner	The relationship between advocate and partner may create a relationship of dependency and still reflects relationships of power
	The independence from services can give the advocate a strong voice	Citizen advocacy schemes tend to be expensive to run and maintain
Peer advocacy	Advocates tend to have had similar experiences, especially of service provision	Advocates' experience may not always be relevant to the partner's experience
	Advocate and partner can have shared experience of surviving and using services	
	Advocate is independent of the service provider and can be supported by a service survivor/user group	Service providers may attempt to disempower peer advocacy as they disempower service users themselves
	Relationships between advocate and partner can be mutual and develop into meaningful friendships	
Professional advocacy	Trained, paid and qualified advocate acting with their partner	Advocates could be in danger of pushing their own agenda rather than the views of people they represent

(Continued)

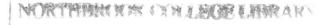

TABLE 5.1   *(CONTINUED)*

Types of advocacy	Characteristics	Weaknesses
Professional advocacy (*Cont.*)	Independent from services or social care organisations	Professional advocates may reflect the needs of service providers to fund advocacy
	Funded from sources away from service providers so that their independence is not compromised	Professional advocates may move on to other employment and leave people in a vacuum
	The professional advocate can be hosted within another community service such as Citizens Advice Bureau or within its own separate organisation	Confirms positions of professional power and expert
	The professional advocate has the backing of an independent organisation and is accountable to the organisation as well as the person	
Parent/carer advocacy	Obligation, care and kinship define the relationship and parents and carers may have the best interest of people at heart	Parents' and carers' needs may override the needs of people who need to have their voices heard
		Possible conflict of interest between the needs of carers and the views of people
		Possible overprotection issues and denial of risk taking
Self-advocacy	People voicing their own views either collectively in groups or individually	May require support from other people
	Challenges professional power and expertise	Requires support from professionals and agencies who may limit the impact of self-advocacy

Source: Based on Goodley and Ramacharan (2005)

The different approaches to advocacy have a range of weaknesses yet it is a central theme of services, especially with people who use learning difficulty services.

Goodley and Ramcharan (2005) also suggest that advocacy has shifted from being led by professionals to being supported by professionals. This has led to a rise in self-advocacy as a model of empowering people. Workers at People First (Open University, 1996) define self-advocacy as speaking up for yourself, being able to stand up for your rights and making choices. For self-advocacy to be a successful empowering process professionals and organisations need to support fully the ethos of self-advocacy and be prepared to have their power challenged and to relinquish the power they have. As Aspis (1999) points out, people in self-advocacy groups should have more power than those advising them and challenge the imbalances of power between disabled and non-disabled people.

People also need to develop the skills they need to advocate for themselves and others yet there are problems in who defines the skills that people need. Agencies and professionals tend to define what is an accepted method of communication rather than accept that different people have different methods of speaking up for themselves.

Aspis (1997; 1999) is critical of how organisations and society have reacted to the self-advocacy movement. She comments that self-advocacy groups have successfully campaigned for moral rights; that is, what people should have. Moral rights are different from legal rights. Legal rights are enforceable while the granting of moral rights is dependent on the goodwill of those in power. As a consequence there is no sanction against those that fail to uphold the moral rights requested by self-advocacy groups.

Aspis (1997) also suggests that self-advocacy groups are in danger of becoming mechanisms for service user consultation rather than challenging the provision of services. Such a method of empowering people reflects a managerial approach rather than a democratic approach. Beresford and Croft (2003) point out that a democratic approach would lead to user-controlled services and a redistribution of power from service providers and professionals to service users. A managerial approach on the other hand maintains a provider-led approach to service delivery.

Service providers can also set the agenda for the scope and influence of self-advocacy. Advocates can speak up, tell their social care worker what they want, tell the Social Services Department how services should look, but those in power can choose to ignore or dismiss the requests of groups and individuals as being inappropriate or unrealistic.

Any concessions made to self-advocacy groups or individuals could be limited and do not challenge the organisation or power of the professional. For advocacy to work real concessions of power are needed.

Social model of disability – a rights model of empowerment

The social model of disability reflects a more democratic approach to empowerment with its aim being user control of services.

An individual or medical model of disability regards an individual's impairment as being responsible for the limitations the individual faces in the world.

Oliver (1981) suggests that it is the physical and social environment which imposes limitations upon people. It is the failure of the social and physical environment to recognise the needs and rights of disabled people.

Activity

Consider the notion that people are disabled by society.
  Describe how society might disable:

o People with learning difficulties or with mental health problems
o People with different cultural and ethnic backgrounds
o Men or Women.

For Swain et al. (1993; 1998; 2004) people encounter disabling barriers which disable them. The barriers are not just the physical ones associated with access to buildings or transport. They are within the organisations and institutions of society, the language and culture we experience that reflects society's attitude towards people and the organisation and delivery of services. These disabling barriers are seen as barriers that oppress people and deny them their rights to be full members of society. Disabling barriers affect people's civil, social, political and moral rights. Underlying this is Swain et al.'s (1998) SEAwall of institutional discrimination (see Figure 5.1) that prevents disabled people from fully participating in society as full and active citizens.

The underpinning of the SEAwall is the *structural level*. The structures of society reflect hierarchical structures of power and dominant ideologies. A view of normality is sustained by the structures of society and organisations which marginalise disabled people and exclude people from society and is linked to poverty and wider inequalities such as access to employment, services and employment. These structural barriers result in people being denied political, social and human rights.

The *environmental level* is about the interface between individuals and the physical and social environment. So these are not only the barriers faced by disabled people in terms of physical access to buildings and public transport, but also the barriers to information through Braille, appropriate signs and symbols (e.g. MAKATON) or interpreters.

The *attitudinal level* is characterised by the personal prejudices of individuals who may hold stereotypical views of disabled people. This becomes an issue

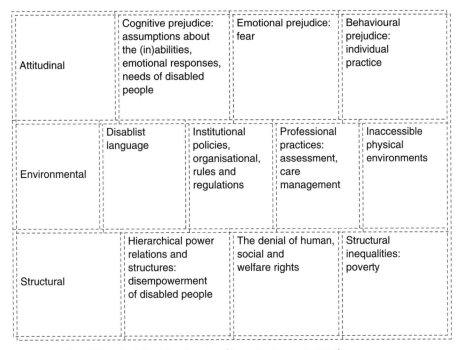

Attitudinal	Cognitive prejudice: assumptions about the (in)abilities, emotional responses, needs of disabled people	Emotional prejudice: fear	Behavioural prejudice: individual practice	
Environmental	Disablist language	Institutional policies, organisational, rules and regulations	Professional practices: assessment, care management	Inaccessible physical environments
Structural	Hierarchical power relations and structures: disempowerment of disabled people	The denial of human, social and welfare rights	Structural inequalities: poverty	

Figure 5.1   *The SEAwall of disabling barriers (from Swain et al., 1998)*

when professionals in positions of power hold prejudicial attitudes towards disabled people, which results in discriminatory and oppressive practice.

The oppression of disabled people is maintained through what sociologists term the dominant ideology. Ideology can be regarded as the values and beliefs of a specific social group. The dominant ideology is the ideas, values and beliefs of the most powerful groups in society. It is these ideas that are transmitted through our cultural heritage, through the media, our newspapers, television and other forms of mass communication, and are taken as common-sense ideas or what is seen as normal and what is seen as abnormal. It is through this transmission of ideas of what is normal that people, who do not fit into the normal, experience disabling barriers. The disabling barriers locate a person's impairment within the individual rather than society, and so the cure for being abnormal is located within the person rather than society.

So as social care and health practitioners, are we reinforcing the oppression of people by confirming and maintaining the disabling barriers? Do we see the answer to disability within the framework of what is normal and are our services based upon what we see people need because it is normal to do so?

As social care workers we are responding to the needs of people who require our services (see Chapter 9). This is undertaken under the umbrella of empowering people who use our services. Yet how far do organisations and practitioners empower people within a framework of tackling disabling barriers?

A model of empowerment based upon the social model of disability is concerned with the breaking down of disabling barriers and the promotion of people's rights. Service users are seen as experts of their own situation and people are regarded as equal and in control of the services that are delivered.

In taking account of the social model of disability Swain et al. (1998) suggest that practitioners need to be aware of disability issues and the factors that create institutional discrimination. This means being aware of the attitudes and behaviour of others and ourselves and the wider structural reasons for the exclusion and marginalisation of disabled people. So as practitioners we need to be aware of how our practice may reinforce disabling barriers. We need to use our professional power to promote rights and so it does not reflect disabling barriers.

Continuum of empowerment

Martin and Henderson (2001) present a four-stage continuum of participation which can be used to locate a service's commitment to empowerment.

At one end is the idea that people have *information* about the services that they receive. The next point on the continuum is *consultation* where people and service user groups can be asked about the services being provided. Consultations with people can be acted upon or ignored by those doing the consulting. Working in *partnership* involves service users being part of the decision-making process and being members of relevant policy-making bodies. Partnerships tend to contain a relationship of power and service users may find themselves in unequal partnerships. *Delegated control* implies giving authority and resources to service user groups to plan and develop user-run services. Delegated services are still accountable to the funding authority.

We would argue that a fifth model could be added to the continuum whereby service users are in total control of services and able to plan and develop services and employ staff to meet their needs (Figure 5.2).

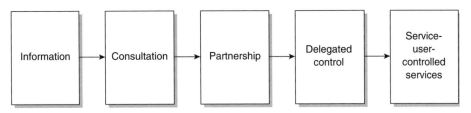

Figure 5.2   The five stage continuum of participation (adapted from Martin and Henderson, 2001)

Activity

Locating your practice on the continuum of empowerment

Using the models of empowerment we have explored and the continuum of empowerment, attempt to locate your practice and service provision on the continuum.

How does your service:

o Give accessible information to people about the services it provides?
o Consult in a meaningful way with people?
o Regard people as equal partners in service provision?
o Delegate part of its service provision to people who use the service?
o Reflect the idea that people should be in charge of the service?

Influence of postmodernism

The rise and influence of postmodernist social theory has not been lost on the notion that moral principles and values should guide our practice. Postmodernist social theory suggests that there is no one truth or overall explanation of the social and human world. Instead there are many truths open to subjective interpretation.

Hugman (2003) explains the postmodernist influences on values in social care. He points out that from the perspective of Foucault, to act ethically is not to deceive and to take as a starting point not to deceive oneself. So it becomes important to scrutinise oneself and be aware of one's own perspectives. Bauman (1994, quoted in Hugman, 2003), another influential postmodernist theorist, suggests that to act morally is to take responsibility for another person and that person's wellbeing is a 'precious thing' that should be preserved and enhanced.

Postmodernism challenges the view that professionals have the answers based upon the theories and ideas that underpin practice. Postmodernist ideas would suggest that there is no certainty in that what we do will result in the outcome that we are hoping to achieve as social care practitioners.

This challenge to professional knowledge also questions the idea of professional power and the view of the professional as the expert. These ideas to some extent tie in with the radical agenda and the views of the disability rights movement.

This postmodern approach to ethics reflects Husband's (1995) ideas of being morally active and the notion of acting as an 'autonomous moral agent'. The postmodernist approach views universal principles as restrictive. It becomes important for practitioners to take moral responsibility for their actions and actively to analyse or reflect on their interventions in people's lives within a moral context.

Postmodernist approaches also remind us that it is important to recognise the position of power that practitioners are in.

Postmodernism is not without its critics (see Hugman, 2003) but it has clearly influenced social care practice, the most significant being to challenge the notion that as social care professionals we need prescriptive codes of practice to guide our actions and interventions in people's lives. What is needed is a framework that may enable practitioners to reflect upon their interventions within a moral context so that as practitioners we can be morally responsible for our actions.

A practice model for working with values

As we have seen, working with values in our practice is a complex yet fundamental part of health and social care practice. For students embarking on their career in health and social care this may create more confusion and dilemmas rather than clarify what is the right way to practise.

Rather than having a prescriptive set of values and moral principles or codes of ethics it is important to take the moral responsibility for your practice. This may seem daunting, even scary, but recognising this is part of the process.

Drawing on Husband's (1995) idea of the morally active practitioner, both Dawson and Butler (2003) and Hugman (2003) have proposed a framework to guide ethical decision making. Using these suggestions as a background and a central value of empowerment it is possible to outline a framework of ethical ideas that you will need to guide your practice. Such a framework can help you as a health and social care practitioner work in the complex area of making ethical decisions that affect people's lives.

To guide your ethical decision making there are things that you need to do:

- **Values:** You need to be aware of your values and moral principles and what you believe in. How do your moral principles fit in with the moral principles that have been explored in this chapter? Can you stay true to your values or do you need to alter your moral perspective and how? Do your beliefs and values reflect the dominant ideology?

- **Ethical conflicts:** You need to be aware of the ethical issues that arise in your practice. This means being explicit about the ethical dilemmas and moral conflicts that you may face when making decisions that affect the people you work with. You need to be aware of and identify the values that exist at different levels and that people have different and diverse ethical principles. Once you have recognised the contradictions and conflicts that exist, you can use this to inform your decision making.

- **Power and empowerment and rights:** Are you aware of power in your relationship with people who use services? Where does the power lie? Are you able to work in an empowering way that reflects people's rights? Does your practice reflect the dominant ideology? Can you enable people to have a say, make decisions about their lives, be in control?

- **Being reflective:** It is important to reflect upon your practice and decision-making process. This process not only enables you to identify values and the ethical issues that you face, but also enables you to learn and develop your practice.

- **Develop a cultural awareness:** You need to be culturally aware and develop your cultural competence (Papadopoulos, 2003). It is also important to recognise and engage in debates concerning multi- and interculturalism.

- **Taking risks:** As a practitioner making ethical decisions you need to be prepared to take risks. Taking risks based on your ethical judgement may bring with it feelings of apprehension. It is important to recognise this as the responsibility for your decision making is yours.

- **Being morally active:** As a practitioner in health and social care you are intervening in people's lives; your practice is a moral activity. You need to be able to work as a morally active practitioner. Be aware of the constraints upon your practice but do let these restrain your practice. Make ethical decisions based upon your moral principles, take responsibility for them and do what you believe is the right thing.

SUMMARY

This chapter has explored the values and moral principles that should underpin your practice. It is important to understand these issues as social care is a moral activity and when we intervene in people's lives we need to do the right thing. We have suggested that there should be a central value of empowerment based on rights with people being in control of their services and the decisions that affect their lives. We have also presented a practice model for working with values stressing the importance of empowering practice and working as a morally active practitioner.

Further reading

Beckett, C. and Maynard, A. (2005) *Values and Ethics in Social Work: An introduction*. London: Sage. This is a readable text which introduces students to values and ethics and manages to bridge the gap between theory and practice.

Cuthbertson, S. and Quallington, J. (2007) *Values for Care Practice*. Newton Abbot: Reflect Press. This book applies values to practice in health and social care and enables students to analyse their own value base.

Acknowledgment

Figure 5.1: This material first appeared in *Confronting Disabling Barriers: Towards Making Organisation Accessible* (1988: Swain, J; Gillman, M; French, S.) published by Venture Press and reproduced by kind permission of the British Association of Social Workers.

6 THE LEGAL AND ORGANISATIONAL CONTEXT OF HEALTH AND SOCIAL CARE

Graham Brotherton

SUMMARY CHAPTER CONTENTS

- Government in the UK
- The history of health and care services
- The current legal and organisational structures of health and social care services
- The broader debate around the 'mixed economy of welfare' and the role of markets in providing health and social care services
- The changing roles of workers and the move towards new models of regulation

---

Learning outcomes

By the end of this chapter, you should be able to:

- Understand the broad structures and systems of government in the UK.

- Appreciate the history of services and how this has influenced current practice.

- Develop your understanding of the centrality of the mixed economy as introduced in Chapter 4.

- Understand how the regulatory structures of health and social care are changing and the importance of this.

The structure of government in the UK

In this chapter we will be looking at the broader legal and organisational context of health and social care. In order to do this it is first necessary to look at how government is structured and the implications that this has for governments in terms of how legislation and policy are developed both generally and in the context of health and social care.

One of the key features of the UK government is that it is very centralised, even allowing for the recent impact of devolution (see later section). This means that the government in general and the prime minister in particular has considerable power and the ability to exert considerable influence on policy. There are a number of overlapping reasons for this. In part this stems from the way in which the government is elected. The 'first past the post' system in which Members of Parliament (MPs) are elected on the basis of who gets the greatest number of votes in a geographical constituency means that effectively government will almost always come from one of two parties, Labour or Conservative. This gives the leaders of these two parties considerable power within the party as effectively political careers are dependent upon being successful within party hierarchies. This is reinforced especially in government by the fact that the leader/prime minister (with close colleagues/advisers) has considerable power of patronage: that is, the ability to appoint people to positions both within government and in 'Quangos' (see box below).

Governments of all political persuasions have been accused of appointing people whose views support the governments to significant roles on 'Quangos', though in the last few years there has been a move to a more open selection process, through advertising for suitable applicants.

Quangos

'Quasi Non-Governmental Organisations' is a term used to refer to a range of organisations that are linked to government (often by funding) but are not technically part of government. There are a number in health and social care, such as the Social Care Institute for Excellence or the Healthcare Commission, which are described later in this chapter.

Activity

Find out about the role of the above organisations (the web addresses can be found later in the chapter). How do they contribute to setting and evaluating the health and social care agenda?

- The use of Quangos to implement policy is not without its critics who high-
- light the fact that they are not directly accountable to either local or national
- electorates in the way that governments or local authorities are.

There are three main elements to central government, the Executive, the Legislature and the Judiciary. The Executive consists of those who have decision-making power, namely the prime minister, the Cabinet Ministers and those who advise them. In policy terms this is where policy tends to be initiated, i.e. where 'ideas' about new policy tend to come from.

The Legislature consists of the two Houses of Parliament, the Commons and the Lords. This is where policy – especially that which requires changes in the law – is discussed or 'debated' and sometimes amended. All potential legislation has to go through a series of readings in the two Houses and also through a series of committee stages where it is scrutinised in more detail by a committees of MPs. While this process does lead to some changes, it is important to note the government can still exert considerable influence because it chooses the timetable for the readings and the composition of the committees which scrutinise the legislation.

The Judiciary contains the senior judges who play a role in terms of defining the way in which legislation 'works' in practice; the Gloucestershire judgment described later in this chapter is an example of this.

It is important to note that to a very considerable extent a government's ability to initiate a push-through legislation is dependent upon the size of its majority in Parliament. The larger the majority, the easier it is to maintain control of the process outlined above. Over the past 25 years or so governments have for most of the time enjoyed sizeable majorities and have therefore been able to push through radical change if they wished to.

The 'traditional' view of the policy process is that governments start the process by putting out a consultation document in the form of a Green Paper which organisations are then able to respond to. Green Papers often include a range of options that are then either proceeded with or dropped on the basis of the response from interested parties. This is followed by a White Paper that tends to set out more definite proposals. After the consultation on the White Paper the government will produce draft legislation, a 'bill' that then enters the process described previously. At the end of this process the bill becomes a new piece of legislation or Act. To give one recent example of this process which has had significant implications for health and social care, in 2003 the government issued a Green Paper on the future of services for children in the light of the report into the death of Victoria Climbie; it was called 'Every Child Matters'. After going through the process described above this became the basis for the Children Act 2004. The introduction of the legislation also illustrates another aspect of the process, as at the time of writing (spring 2007) there are still major consultation documents being produced about the implementation of the Act and several important aspects of the Act will not be implemented until 2008. In cases such as this where changes are far-reaching and significant, the consultation process over the detail of fully implementing new policy/legislation may go on for several years.

It is, though, important to highlight that not all new policy follows this route: some changes do not require changes in the law and are brought about by government changing the advice/'instructions' it gives to local or NHS authorities in the form of policy guidance. A change in the way funding is provided or targeted can also be used to change the direction of policy. While the role of local authorities in direct service provision is declining, they remain significant as commissioners of services. This process of utilising the mixed economy as a basis for policy and using non-governmental agencies as a key element of policy implementation has been described as a shift away from government to a broader framework of governance. There is a good summary of how the process of introducing legislation works as well as useful information on many other aspects of government at http://www.parliament.uk/works/works.cfm.

Devolution

One of the key changes of the last few years has been the introduction of devolution, which has led to the creation of a Scottish Parliament and Welsh Assembly and the transfer of powers to this 'new' tier of government. In the case of the Scottish Parliament this includes full responsibility for health and social care issues. In the case of the Welsh Assembly there is a greater overlap with the UK Parliament but policy in Wales is clearly diverging in some areas.

From a policy point of view, one of the most interesting implications of devolution is the emergence of different emphases and approaches to health and social care policy within the different parts of the UK. At present, perhaps this is most pronounced in the area of policy around children, e.g. the differing roles of the Children's Commissioners in England, Scotland and Wales (and Northern Ireland). There are, though, a range of other issues as illustrated in relation to charging policies for both prescriptions and social care services.

Activity

If your role involves working with children, you may find it useful to explore the three Children's Commissioners web sites which can be easily found through any search engine. Look at the differences in roles and emphases between the different commissioners. What might explain these differences in emphases between the three roles?

Local government

In Scotland and Wales, the structure of local authorities is quite straightforward with a system of 'unitary' authorities, a single layer of local government where all have the same roles and responsibilities. In the case of England the system (largely for historical reasons as reform has been incremental) is more complex; some areas of England (mainly the large urban areas) have unitary authorities, whereas other areas have a two-tier system of district and county councils. In this case responsibility for health and social care lies with the county authority. The role of local authorities in the provision of social care has changed significantly with a move away from direct provision towards a purchasing and co-ordination role, though there are still considerable variations in the amount of direct provision between local authorities.

Activity

- Relevant current consultation documents can be found on the relevant government departments web sites (Department of Health, Department for Children, Schools and Families (DCSF), Scottish Executive, Welsh Assembly). Have a look at any relevant consultation documents.
- If there are any that are particularly relevant to your area of interest, think about whether you might want to respond individually, as a student group or as a group of work colleagues.

Implementing policy

In implementing policy, governments have a number of 'levers' in terms of ensuring that policy 'works' in the way that was intended. The first is finance. Central government provides the bulk of the money which local authorities use to provide services and often this is given in ways so that it has to be used in particular ways through targeted funding, which can only be used for specific purposes. A second way in which central government is able to control policy is through using legislation to create 'statutory duties', which are things that local authorities must do, e.g. providing a child protection service.

A third option open to central government is to give local authorities 'powers' which are the ability to undertake particular functions. Much of the Community Care legislation works in this way and it gives local authorities greater discretion. However, in may cases the use of 'powers' is clarified by the production of guidance, which may in itself create a fairly tight framework within which agencies have to operate (see for example the discussion on Community Care Assessments in Chapter 9). The final major 'tool' available to government is the use of inspectorates such as the Commission for Social Care

Inspection or Ofsted to scrutinise services; this is discussed in more detail in a later section.

The development of health and social care services

In order to understand the current structure of health and social care services, it is helpful to give a brief history of the development of services. This is inevitably a brief overview and for more detail you might want to look at the history chapters in the recommended texts at the end of the chapter. A more detailed account can be found in Fraser's fascinating history of the development of welfare in the UK.

The nineteenth century

The government started to become significantly involved in welfare in the nineteenth century through the Poor Law Reform Act of 1834. This is best remembered now as the piece of legislation which introduced the 'workhouse' system under which the only form of assistance available to people in poverty was to enter the workhouse, an institution systematically designed to be as unpleasant as possible in order to deter all but the 'genuinely' destitute. The legacy of this system has had a major influence on the development of health and care services in several ways. Firstly, one of the consequences of the poor law system as it developed was the recognition of the need for some form of (fairly rudimentary) health care system. This lead to the development of the 'Poor Law Infirmaries' which grew up in the latter part of the nineteenth century. The Poor Law Infirmaries tended to be poorly staffed – often with virtually no medical presence – and were often overcrowded. Reports from the time suggest that the quality of care was also very variable. However the Poor Law Infirmaries were later to become a central part of the NHS at its inception (of which more later).

A second way in which the workhouse had an impact was that the population of the workhouses tended to consist predominantly of those with few other options: older people, those with disabilities, those who might now be perceived as having acute mental health conditions and women who had become pregnant outside of marriage. As a consequence, in many cases the workhouses soon reached capacity. There were two responses to this. One was an attempt to categorise the workhouse population and develop other institutions to provide for those that 'needed' it. This was a key factor in the growth of the mental health and learning disability institutions in particular and the placement in those institutions of large numbers of women under the catch-all category of 'moral defective'. A 'flavour' of life in the workhouse can be found on the National Trust web site in respect of the workhouse at Southwell.

The second response was quite different: this was the emergence of charitable organisations. Many of the big charities which still exist today, such as Barnardo's, The National Society for the Prevention of Cruelty to Children (NSPCC) and its Scottish equivalent, the SSPCC, have their 'roots' in this period as did 'Cottage Hospitals'. They emerged partly because the workhouses, especially in urban areas, were unable to respond adequately to the prevalence of poverty, but crucially in many cases because of the moral or ethical beliefs of those who set them up. These were predominantly associated with particular non-conformist Christian groups such as Methodists or Quakers. By the later part of the nineteenth century these many and varied charitable organisations were providing more 'poor relief' as most welfare was at this time categorised than the 'state' system based on the workhouse. There are very useful sections on some of the charities' web sites which give a clear picture of their development; see for example the history section on the Barnardo's web site.

As much of the charity was based on a moral perspective, there was a perceived need to ensure that assistance was given to the deserving poor. A group emerged which tried to give charitable giving a clearer structure to ensure that the above aim was met, namely the Charity Organisation Society or COS founded in 1869. The COS pioneered a way of working based on 'casework', the systematic collection of facts about an individual's or family's circumstances to ensure that resources were given to the most needy and deserving. This model of casework has remained a central underpinning of approaches to care work, especially social work, ever since, right through to current models of care management (see Chapter 9).

A further consequence of this model was to ensure that those who were not seen as deserving, namely unmarried mothers, those characterised as feckless, etc., found it even more difficult to access help, thus tying them to the workhouse and its successor institutions.

The creation of the 'welfare state'

By the end of the nineteenth century there was increasing pressure for reform, partly from elements within the charitable movement but also from organisations such as the growing trade union movement and the political party that this produced – the Labour Party. In addition elements within the Liberal Party, at this stage a much more significant party than Labour, also recognised the need for change. In 1906 this combination of factors leads to the election of a Liberal government with support from the Labour Party. Over the next few years this government introduced a series of measures which are still recognisable as the basis of our existing system: old age pensions, school meals, legislation against child neglect and the introduction of National Insurance to fund a limited benefit system and the first attempt at systematic health care (at least for male workers), the 'panel doctor' system. These were all introduced between 1906 and 1912. By 1912 the focus shifted to international issues with the impending First World War and whilst the post-war Liberal government did introduce some reform, notably by giving local authorities extended powers to build houses, the system remained fundamentally similar until the start of the Second World War.

During the Second World War the government commissioned a senior civil servant, William Beveridge, to look at the technical workings of the benefit system. Beveridge's report somewhat exceeded his brief and called for wholesale reform of the whole welfare system, arguing that the interconnected nature of the problems associated with poverty, unemployment, etc., required an interconnected response. The Beveridge Report, 'Social Insurance and Allied Services', published in 1942 was effectively a blueprint for a welfare state and formed the basis for the general election at the end of the Second World War with the Labour Party promising to implement Beveridge in full and the Conservatives largely opposed. The only aspect of Beveridge which was implemented before the election were the proposals for education which formed the basis for the 1944 Education Act with its introduction of a unified system of grammar and secondary modern schools that have shaped all subsequent education policy.

The post-war election resulted in a landslide victory for Labour, the first time the party had enjoyed an overall majority in Parliament, and the Beveridge proposals now became the basis of far-reaching social reform in health, benefits and the personal social services. In part the NHS had already come into existence as the Wartime Health Service, a co-ordinated system set up to meet the demands of war. It was not popular with many within the medical profession for a number of reasons, both financial and professional, and the concessions offered by the Health Secretary, Anuerin Bevan, to persuade the medical profession to join the NHS, in which doctors remained independent contractors within the NHS rather than employees, have had long-lasting consequences (see the section on NHS reform). When the NHS was formally set up in 1948 it marked a decisive shift, giving women and children full access to health care for the first time, setting up a proper primary care system through the General Practitioner system and integrating the various strands of hospital provision, the teaching hospitals, the cottage hospitals, the municipal hospitals (which the Poor Law Infirmaries had become), into a coherent whole. The NHS was a hugely popular innovation, a status it was to maintain for the next 30 years or so. However it also proved much more expensive than had been anticipated: costs doubled in the first two years and there was no 'peak' as some had anticipated (that costs would be high at first but would fall as people became healthier as a result of the NHS and consequently costs would fall). Managing the cost of the NHS rapidly became a political issue that has endured right through to the present.

In the social care area the government set up both Welfare Departments for adults and Children's Departments, marking the first time that the state had become significantly involved in provision in this area – many of the services which now form the mainstream of social care provision such as residential care and child protection were introduced at this time. The Children's and Welfare Departments were merged into generic Social Services Departments in 1970.

Perhaps the most significant of the Beveridge proposals were these for the restructuring of the benefit system, which proved to have ramifications that have influenced the whole of subsequent policy development. Beveridge proposed a contributory system based on National Insurance in which workers would pay in while in work and receive while not working (providing that they had paid sufficient contributions). Women would pay contributions while working, but as they left the workforce upon marriage they would then receive access to benefits through their husband. Beveridge anticipated that as there was a return to near full employment after the war, the system would become largely self-funding.

For those who were unable to access the contributory scheme, a safety net scheme called National Assistance was introduced. This was intended to be a minor part of the system, but for a complex variety of reasons, e.g. the fact that there was no return to full employment and later that this was the only benefit women not living with their husband could claim, this soon became the larger element of the benefit system. Efforts to control National Assistance and its successors, Supplementary Benefit and Income Support, have been a major feature of social policy right through to New Labour and 'Welfare to Work'.

A central element of the Beveridge plan in the years immediately after the war was housing provision. In the decade immediately after the war two-thirds of all house building was undertaken by local authorities and social housing became a significant part of provision. While there were some significant attempts at reform and reorganisation over the next 20 years, the basis of the Beveridge system remained in place until the late 1970s, though after the recession of the early 1970s spending in some areas, e.g. house building, fell markedly.

The New Right reform

The period after 1979 saw a process of radical reform in a number of areas: in housing the end of local authority house building and the introduction of the opportunity for local authority tenant's to buy the house they lived in. The consequence of this has been the effective removal of housing from the welfare policy area which some critics have argued is currently having a negative impact on the government's ability to deliver 'joined-up' services. This has been partially addressed in recent years through the 'Supporting People' programme which funds housing-related support to enable vulnerable people to remain in independent accommodation (for fuller information see http://www.spkweb. org.uk/).

In benefits, the period saw the introduction of the Income Support System based around fixed levels of payment for people who fall into specific categories, which still exists in amended form. For health and social care, though, the significant change was the implementation in 1990 of the National Health Service and Community Care Act. In order to explore this fully it is important to place this in the context of the debate about the ideological context of health and social care.

The ideological context of health and social care

Health and social care as with other areas of welfare takes place in an ideological context: that is, they are heavily influenced by the political views of the government of the day. The expansion of 'Welfare' between 1945 and 1951 took place in the context of a government committed to social democracy whereas the reforms of the 1980s and early 1990s took place in the context of a New Right (sometimes referred to as 'Thatcherite' after the prime minister of the bulk of this period) approach.

The basis of social democracy is that the state has a positive role to play in the provision of services. This is because in a 'market' context (see next section) services (in our case health, education, etc.) will be allocated on the basis of ability to pay rather than need. This is what social democrats refer to as 'market failure' – in order to ensure fairness the state needs to get involved to ensure all citizens receive adequate support. This is sometimes called 'positive freedom', the idea being that people need positive support from the state in order to be able take advantage of the opportunities that might be available to them. The money needed to provide for these services is raised through taxation. Taxation is also related to income and the ability to pay, so higher earners pay tax at a higher rate. This is referred to as progressive taxation and is linked to a belief that the system should be redistributive, giving on the basis of need.

New Right thinking emerged as a reaction to this. It argued that the inevitable consequence of social democracy was bureaucracy and inefficiency and that the welfare system had a tendency to trap people in dependency on the state. The solution was to reduce the role of the state by reducing its role as a service provider, through the privatisation of services. This would also introduce competition between service providers, leading to greater choice and efficiency, and free up money which could be used to reduce taxes, giving people the opportunity to take greater responsibility for themselves. Of particular significance to the New Right critique has been the way in which public services it is argued tend to be inflexible and unresponsive and to deliver a 'one size fits all' service, rather than one tailored to the specific needs of patients and service users. While in practice even most New Right governments have retained some element of progressive taxation, most are critical of the principle, arguing for a move towards a 'flatter' tax system in which everyone pays the same rate on all income.

Central to New Right thinking is a belief in a 'free market' system, which in this context is a belief that market principles of supply and demand apply even to welfare services, i.e. that if someone 'supplies' a good or service at an appropriate price there will be 'demand' for it: the better the price and quality, the greater the demand. If a good or service is of poor quality or priced too high for its market 'demand' will fall and the supplier will need to adjust price, quality or both in order to become competitive. This leads to the best goods or services being available at the most competitive prices – so-called 'market discipline'. It also leads to flexibility and choice, as there are likely to be a range of providers competing to provide appropriate services. In this model the NHS and social care services could and should be provided in the same way as any other good or service.

There are, however, two key problems in the area of welfare. One is how to introduce market forces into areas where the state is the only or most dominant provider of services. This is dealt with in the next section. The second is the 'problem' of free services, as, in a market model, providing a service free is likely to lead to an excess of demand – of which more later.

New Labour emerged in the 1990s as an attempt to reconcile a commitment to social justice with a belief in markets. Its adherents claimed that it encompassed key features of both social democracy and the New Right, hence the claim to be a new approach – the 'Third Way'. New Labour in government has retained in a modified way most of the market reforms of the 1980s and 1990s but has also developed some distinctively new elements which are explored at the end of this chapter.

The NHS and Community Care Act 1990 is best seen as an attempt to introduce this market approach into health and social care services. There are a number of parallels between the health reforms and the social care reforms, but there were also significant differences, therefore each is dealt with separately.

NHS reform

The NHS prior to reform was a large and monolithic organisation. Reforms in the 1980s had attempted to introduce more 'effective' management but the 1990 changes took things much further. At the heart of the reforms was the so-called 'internal market', an attempt to create market-like structures in the NHS. In order to facilitate this, the NHS needed to be broken up structurally into units that could compete with each other. In addition, in order for the principles of supply and demand to apply there needed to be parts of the NHS which supplied services (providers) and parts which demanded/bought services (purchasers or commissioners). For this reason the reforms were often referred to as introducing the purchaser/provider split.

The purchaser 'organisations' were firstly health authorities, the part of the NHS that had previously dealt with local planning; their role in the new system was to identify likely local demand and to buy services to meet this demand. The second purchasing organisations were 'GP fundholders', GP practices which had opted to take the sum of money which would have been allocated to the health authority to buy services for its patients and to spend it directly on its patients' behalf. Over time the government felt that the role of the health authorities would diminish (and eventually disappear) as more and more GP practices become fundholding.

In order to have a range of possible 'providers' the remainder of the NHS, primarily hospitals and associated services, was broken up into a series of competing 'trusts'. These were of variable size and composition as they emerged from a bidding process, but have become increasingly similar in the intervening period through a process of mergers. NHS trusts were independent organisations with their own management structure of chief executive and board which in their original form were intended to compete with other trusts for the 'business' provided by health authorities and GP fundholders (e.g. common surgical procedures) on the grounds of both price and quality. This was referred to as the internal market.

When the Labour Party was elected in 1997 the system was reorganised again. The NHS trusts were maintained with similar management structures but given a new role as local service providers. The purchaser role was given to a new type of organisation – the primary care trust (PCT) – which over a period of time took over the role of purchasing (now referred to as commissioning) local health services. PCTs now control about 80 per cent of the health budget and either provide directly or commission off other agencies, e.g. GP practices, the bulk of 'front line' health services.

PCTs in turn are accountable to a revised tier of health authorities, now called strategic heath authorities, which have an overall planning and monitoring role.

A useful guide to the complex structure of the NHS and the at times confusing terminology can be found on the NHS web site.

Social care reform

Social care reform has in many senses paralleled NHS reform. The NHS and Community Care Act 1990 also applied to social care, but the reforms took a slightly different form. The 'purchaser' role here was given to Social Services Departments who were to be responsible for a new system of assessment and care management (this process is discussed more fully in Chapter 9) in which individuals who might require assistance were assessed, firstly to see whether they were eligible for services (see the Gloucestershire judgment below) and then to see what their needs were. A financial assessment also took place at the same time to identify whether the person should pay part or all of the cost of the services they require.

> The Gloucestershire judgment was a House of Lords decision in 1996, which clarified the NHS and Community Care Act. It states that local authorities in undertaking community care assessments are able to take into account whether they have sufficient resources to provide a service unless not providing a service would put someone at serious physical risk.

The services that people need were to be provided largely in the private and voluntary sectors. The financial regime that introduced this version of community care forced local authorities into spending money buying services from private and voluntary organisations and they were also encouraged to divest themselves of the residential and related provision that they had. In most cases these were separated from the local authority and set up as independent not-for-profit companies.

Unlike in health care the general structures remained largely unchanged even after 1997, though in some specific areas there have been changes. Perhaps the most significant has been the introduction of the 'Fair Access to Care' approach. Under the previous system local authorities set both eligibility criteria for services and the financial assessment framework locally. This led to considerable variations between authorities in terms of both services provided and charges. As a response the government introduced 'Fair Access to Care', a system of national guidelines in an attempt to introduce greater consistency. This is discussed further in Chapter 9.

The new institutional framework for social care

As part of the reforms of the social care system a number of key new institutions have been introduced, as in the box below.

The General Social Care Council, www.gscc.org.uk

This is the regulatory body for social care workers, which will ultimately register all social care staff, who will all be expected to work in accordance with the code of practice for social care workers, which covers a broad range of practice-related areas. There is also a code of practice for social care employers . If you are not already familiar with the code of practice you might want to look at the GSCC web site now. It also includes the most current information on the timescales for implementation of the registration process.

The Commission for Social Care Inspection, www.csci.org.uk

This is the body that inspects social care services (including the work of Social Services Departments) for all groups and across all sectors. Its reports can be found on the web site as can the national minimum standards for various service user groups which are used as the basis of the inspection process. It has a range of powers that can be used if services are deemed to be substandard up to and including closing services down.

The Social Care Institute for Excellence, www.scie.org.uk

This body has a remit to promote good practice in social care work, through research, consultation and dissemination of good practice. It also hosts the Social Care Online database (see Chapter 2).

There are also a group of parallel institutions in the health sector, as follows.

The Nursing and Midwifery Council, www.nmc-uk.org

This has responsibility for registration and professional practice issues for health care professionals. Unlike the GSCC it does not include registration of those without a 'professional' qualification.

The Healthcare Commission (or legally, The Commission for Healthcare Audit and Inspection), www.chai.org.uk

This has responsibility for the inspection of health services (except for those provided by foundation trusts – which have a separate inspection system), but where services overlap this is carried out in conjunction with the Commission for Social Care Inspection (CSCI).

The National Institute for Health and Clinical Excellence, www.nice.org.uk

This body has a range of activities including licensing the introduction of new treatments, evaluating health interventions and the publication of guidance for professionals on a range of issues. It includes both clinical and public health issues.

Managerialism and surveillance

One way in which the changes of the past 20 years or so have been explained is through the emergence of managerial approaches to health and social care. Managerialism is a set of ideas that emerged from the New Right critique of welfare services and is based on the idea that public services need to be managed in the same way as commercial organisations. There are tensions in managerialism as an approach in that it has tended to highlight both the need for flexibility in service delivery and the need for targets to assess performance/service delivery, with critics suggesting the latter approach has proved dominant. Linked to managerialism has been a distrust of professional autonomy which has led to increased surveillance through the various inspection bodies. (The implications of this are considered in more detail in Chapters 9 and 10.)

Joining up services

Undeniably the most radical part of the New Labour agenda has been the moves to encourage collaboration and in some cases mergers between health and social care agencies. There have been a number of White Papers and associated pieces of legislation; the central focus of all of them has been to promote a multi-agency approach to service delivery. This can be seen right across the health and social care sector, e.g. in the development of children's trusts which will integrate education and care services for children and the move towards care trusts which will integrate health and care services for adults, though there are as yet only a limited number of these.

A further element of the 'joined-up' approach has been the development of National Service Frameworks (NSFs). These are blueprints for the development of services in particular areas which include older people, mental health and children and which actively promote the development of integrated services.

> A list of the current NSFs and brief summaries can be found on the NHS web site. There are also links to the full versions of the frameworks on the Department of Health web site.

Health and social care under New Labour – changed direction or the New Right continued?

One of the central issues when trying to consider the way in which health and social care has developed under New Labour is to what extent is policy a continuation of the New Right reforms of the 1980s and to what extent does it represent a new phase? There is in some senses evidence for both. There is certainly more private sector involvement in the NHS and a strong commitment from government for this to develop further: for example, through the use of private companies to undertake 'routine' operations in health care and the increasing dominance of private providers right across the social care sector. Furthermore, the way in which 'choice' in a market sense has become the mantra for change across this sector has shades of the New Right critique.

However, there has also been a real increase in health spending as a proportion of public spending (though this is less clear cut in social care, especially adult social care). In social care the move towards more privatised and marketised services has been perhaps less publicised and as a consequence less debated.

Two further aspects of the New Labour reforms which warrant mentioning are firstly the use of targeted services to tackle deep-rooted disadvantage and secondly the central importance of work as an aspect of welfare. Targeted services, of which perhaps the most prominent has been the 'Sure Start' programme, are where areas of particular disadvantage with a high concentration of families have received additional funding to provide appropriate services, e.g. childcare or a greater health visitor presence, though there have been other examples, e.g. the 'action zone' approach in health and education. Sure Start also provides an example of the emphasis on employment as one function of the projects has been to provide childcare and training in order to help parents find work. Another example is the so-called 'new deal approach' which includes a specific strand aimed at helping people with disabilities find employment.

What does the future hold?

With the increased emphasis on public sector reform, this suggests that the future in organisational terms for both health and social care agencies is uncertain. The Green Paper on the reform of social care services, *Independence, Wellbeing and Choice* (Department of Health, 2005), and the subsequent White Paper *Our health, our care, our say* (Department of Health, 2006) perhaps give some useful clues. They propose giving people who use care services greater control over the services they receive with a possible move towards a brokerage-based system giving people an individual budget which could be spent with a range of providers. The social work role is likely to be reconfigured in response to the emergence of this brokerage role with an emphasis on linking people with appropriate services which meet their needs (very much as an insurance broker does with insurance products). Whether this role will be completely separate from the assessment process is not yet clear. The Green Paper can therefore be seen as a further development of the current emphasis on choice and the mixed economy.

Responses have been varied: many commentators have seen the Green and White Papers as a welcome move towards the greater empowerment of users of care services; others have suggested that there is too little focus on the 'basics', e.g. the provision of minor home alterations and that to deliver the new approach effectively would require an increase in resources which is not acknowledged in the Green Paper.

Most recent policy announcements and proposals suggest that in the short to medium term, policy is likely to be guided by the same principles as recent reform.

Review questions   ?

As you finish this chapter you might want to think about the following questions:

- To what extent are current patterns of health and care services the product of the historical development of services?
- What role does ideology play in the development of services?
- How likely is the New Labour agenda to deliver better health and care services? Why? What are the strengths and limitations of the current model?

Further reading

Many of sources identified in Chapter 2 would be useful here, especially the various government web sites and the 'trade press'.

One of the main difficulties with policy is that its rapidly changing context means that books tend to date quickly; using journals is therefore important in maintaining a clear view of the current position. The following journals are likely to be particularly helpful:

Journal of Social Policy
Social Policy and Administration
Social Policy and Society

For a historical perspective in clear and highly readable accounts, see:
Fraser, D. (2002) *The Evolution of the British Welfare State*. London: Palgrave Macmillan.
Timmins, N. (2001) *The Five Giants: A Biography of the Welfare State*. London: Harper Collins.
For a fuller exploration of ideological perspectives and how they link to policy, see:
Lavallette, M. and Pratt, A. (2006) *Social Policy: Theories, Concepts and Issues*. London: Sage.
For a clear overview of policy on a more general level, see:
Blakemore, K. (2003) *Social Policy: An Introduction*. Maidenhead: Open University Press.
Bochel, C. et al. (2005) *Social Policy: Issues and Developments*. London: Prentice Hall.
Robert Gordon University provides an excellent social policy web site with lots of useful content. at: http://www2.rgu.ac.uk/publicpolicy/introduction/contents.htm.

7 PSYCHOLOGY FOR HEALTH AND SOCIAL CARE

Nadine Pearce

SUMMARY CHAPTER CONTENTS

- The components of behaviour
- Psychological theories
- Lifespan development
- Psychology and working in health and social care

Learning objectives

By the end of this chapter, you should be able to:

■ Provide a brief explanation of the major psychological perspectives.

■ Give examples of how emotions, cognitive processes and social interactions influence observable behaviour.

■ Identify the changes associated with significant life stages and suggest reasons for possible responses (developmental outcomes).

■ Discuss how selected psychological theory and concepts can be applied to enhance practice in health and social care settings.

Introduction

As you have chosen to study subjects related to working in the field of health and social care you are inevitably going to be interested in people. Working in this area means that you will be involved in helping people manage their lives, meet their needs and support changing behaviours. By understanding psychological processes you will be able to increase your insight into both your own and your client's behaviours, which will allow greater reflection and enhance the care that you provide.

Psychology and components of behaviour

Psychology is defined as the study of human behaviour. It is concerned with how people behave and the influences that are responsible for that behaviour.

When psychologists use the word 'behaviour' they recognise different elements that include:

- Physiological changes
- Emotional responses
- Cognitive (thinking) processes
- Social interactions
- Actions (observable behaviours).

Activity

Think of a behaviour involving stress, and suggest how each of the above elements of your behaviour could be affected. For example, you could use an important hospital appointment or interview.

Examples of changes you may have considered are as follows.

Physiological changes

If you are feeling anxious or hurried then you may feel that your heart is beating faster or that you have 'butterflies in your stomach'. You may notice that you are either pale or flushed and may even find your hands shaking.

Emotional responses

You could feel frightened or worried and either become more likely to cry or get angry.

Cognitive processes

If you are very worried it may be difficult for you to concentrate so that you need to keep checking the information about time or how to get to the appointment.

Drawing on memories and knowledge, you may find yourself trying to predict what will happen in the consultation and rehearsing explanations and questions.

Social

From previous experiences of your own or others you will be able to make assumptions of how both you as a patient and the doctor are expected to behave. This will influence the clothes that you wear and how you speak to the hospital staff.

You may find it reassuring to take a friend or relative with you so that you have the opportunity to share the experience.

Actions

How you act as a result of these processes will vary with the individual. Some may become so anxious that they do not even go to the appointment, while others will be sufficiently familiar with the situation to feel quite calm and be able to give information clearly and ask appropriate questions. You may find yourself being disorganised and arriving late, or having a high need to be in control so that you get to the appointment very early.

Activity

Now think of an example of a client's behaviour that seems unusual or is causing a problem for the client, family or staff.

Under each of the same headings try to suggest alternative influences that could be causing this behaviour. For example:

o What stresses might be causing unusually angry behaviour in a client?
o In what ways could they be showing this anger?
o What could be the effects on their physical health or social relationships?

By recognising the complexity of influences on behaviours, the health and social care worker is able to remain open to alternative contributory factors and be able to help plan effective interventions and strategies. The study of psychology introduces you to how different theorists can explain the causes of behaviour. In the next section you are encouraged to consider how you can apply this knowledge to individual situations and service users with whom you work.

Psychological theories

Psychologists have different approaches to the way that they attempt to explain the causes of behaviour. Some of these are known as 'schools' or theoretical perspectives. Early psychologists believed that it would be possible to develop a single theory that could explain all aspects of behaviour, but we now realise that human behaviour is so complex, and there are so many different influences, that this may never be possible. However, the different approaches have all contributed to our understanding of how people behave and why. The major theoretical approaches include:

- Physiological approaches
- Learning theories
- Developmental cognitive theory
- Psychodynamic psychology
- Humanistic theories
- Ecological theory.

Physiological approaches

This approach examines how behaviour is determined by heredity and the body's structure and functioning. You are probably aware of how your physical state can also affect your mood, ability to manage your life and your susceptibility to illness.

Some of these influences on development and personality will originate from before birth:

- Genes and chromosomes are inherited from both parents. This will determine whether you are male or female, the colour of your eyes and skin, and whether you will be susceptible to some diseases, e.g. sickle cell anaemia and cystic fibrosis. It sometimes happens that following fertilisation there can be faulty cell division which may lead to genetic disorders such as Down's syndrome.

- During prenatal development the foetus may be exposed to substances that can harm it, including drugs, infections or lack of important nutrients or oxygen.
- Birth experiences, including premature or difficult births, may also affect later development.

Other influences appear after birth, and relate to the speed and nature of maturation. For example, sometimes a baby is born with teeth while others will not start to get any until they are over a year old. Equally some families have a tendency towards greying hair, early or late onset of puberty or menopause.

Developmental charts are based on the recognition that there is a 'normal' or average time when maturational stages occur. These are used to check that milestones in a child's development are consistent to the expected range. There will be considerable variation in rates of development but if a child does not seem to be following the anticipated pattern the child would be monitored more closely or have investigations made. If developmental problems, such as restricted growth syndrome or deafness, are noticed early, interventions can be started that will help improve the chances of the child reaching his or her potential.

Nature or nurture?

The extent to which people are influenced by their inherited characteristics formed part of a major issue for developmental psychologists known as the Nature v. Nurture debate. This was an attempt to try to identify the effect of genetic inheritance compared with the experiences that children are exposed to as they grow up.

The genetic inheritance that you are born with is known as the genotype, and how this is actually realised is the phenotype. A child may be born with a gene for height, but detrimental effects of disease or diet might result in the child not growing very tall. Similarly, if you are born with the ability to learn to talk but never hear anyone speaking you are unlikely to be able to speak a language fluently. However, it is more difficult to separate genetic inheritance and environmental influence in other behaviours such as intelligence, obesity or special skills such as music.

Some psychologists are particularly interested in how genes contribute to the development of personality, suggesting that inborn temperaments will affect how we interact with others including carers. Being born either shy or emotionally reactive, placid or restless, could affect how others respond to us, which could impact on the way that we are accepted or 'fit in' with others' expectations of how we 'should' behave.

The key issue for this debate is the recognition of how inherited characteristics interact with environmental experiences in contributing to development and behaviours.

CASE STUDY

Elsa's parents both describe themselves as shy. They moved to this country before she was born but have not made many new friends.

Elsa has always been content to stay at home and play but her parents are anxious that she should learn to mix and not be shy with other children. They took her to a toddler group and now at 3 years old she has started playgroup. However, Elsa seems unhappy and rather frightened of the more boisterous children. In discussion with the playgroup supervisor it has been agreed that Elsa would get to the hall early so that she had chance to settle in before the others arrive. An allocated play leader would spend time with Elsa starting with quiet activities and then gradually moving further into the centre of the room. After a few weeks Elsa seems much more settled and although she still does not take part in some of the noisier activities, she is at times willing to play without the presence of 'her special play leader'. It is hoped that through these experiences she will continue to gain in confidence and develop friendships to help with her transition to school in two years' time.

Learning theories

Behaviourist approaches

Learning theorists focus on how behaviour is changed as a result of environmental experience, with the concentration on observable behaviour rather than mental processes. This has led to the development of two explanations of learning:

- Classical conditioning
- Operant conditioning.

Classical conditioning is based on the work of Ivan Pavlov who identified that biological responses could become associated with a previously neutral stimulus. Food brings about salivation but learning makes you salivate to familiar ice cream jingles. Likewise, feelings of nausea can result from the smell of a food that has previously caused severe sickness.

THEORY BOX

'LEARNING TO BE FRIGHTENED'

Classical conditioning theorists such as Pavlov believed that phobias (a form of extreme and irrational anxiety about a situation or object) can be acquired by conditioning. This type of learning can be very resistant to change and can form an important part of apparently illogical or habitual behaviours.

Children who have learnt to associate doctors or dentists with pain may still experience a fear of visiting them in adulthood even when they know that no pain will be involved.

Operant conditioning focuses on how behaviour is shaped by its outcome. If there is a pleasurable outcome then it is more likely to be repeated in the future. These good outcomes, described as reinforcers, may be either when something pleasant happens such as praise, attention, money or 'brownie points' or where something unpleasant stops happening, e.g. when a headache improves after taking a tablet.

Conditioning is widely used in both social and educational settings. Examples of how it can be used include developing a programme to help someone recover their mobility or for a child to alter his or her disruptive behaviour.

It is necessary to be very clear about:

• What is the existing behaviour, i.e. the starting point.
• The hoped-for change or goal.
• The steps needed to reach that goal.
• The reinforcer.

The reinforcer must be significant for that person and the steps towards the goal achievable so that they can be rewarded (Figure 7.1).

In everyday life it can be difficult to be clear about what behaviours are being reinforced and it may not be the ones that are expected; it is also very common to try to be too general and aim at modifying too many behaviours at the same time.

Activity

Six-year-old John is considered a difficult pupil. In his class students work in small groups and are expected to remain in their seats when working at activities but John is always getting up and wandering around other tables interfering with their work or chatting. When he approaches the other children they

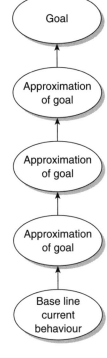

Figure 7.1 *Reinforcers given on successfully achieving each approximation of the goal*

- can get cross at him and may shout or cry. The teacher may also tell him off, and will usually take him back to his table and talk to him about his work, therefore trying to get him to focus on the activity.
- What do you think the teacher is hoping will be the reinforcement for John?
- What might the teacher actually be reinforcing which will increase the likelihood that he will continue with his disruptive behaviour?

In this situation it is possible that attention is the important reinforcer for John, so it is his disruptive behaviours rather than quiet activities that are being reinforced.

Learned helplessness

According to Seligman (1975), another consequence of conditioning can be that we learn what we cannot do. In situations when people believe that they have little or no control they may initially react by increasing effort to find ways of managing the situation, described as a stage of reactance. However, if despite all their efforts they still feel powerless then they have learnt that it is not possible to succeed and give up trying.

Learned helplessness has also been associated with depression as both are characterised by apathy and a low belief in the ability to control situations.

C A S E   S T U D Y

Rita had been successfully managing at home but has recently had a few falls causing a fracturing of her wrist. This made it difficult for her to take care of herself so she agreed to move into a residential care setting. Rita settled in well apart from a worry that due to urgency incontinence she needed to be able to get to the toilet quickly.

Due to concerns about the risk of falling, Rita was advised to ring for help when she wanted to go to the toilet. However, it was not always possible for Rita to get help immediately, so to avoid problems she would try to walk to the toilet on her own.

As this behaviour was seen as a risk, Rita's room was reorganised making it difficult for her to get out of her chair without help. After a few times when she was incontinent, because she was not able to get help quickly enough, it was recommended that she wore an incontinent pad to avoid getting distressed.

Within a few weeks Rita had become incontinent and made no effort to use the toilet.

PRACTICE TIPS

When developing a client's care plans consider:

- How the programme is designed to be specific to that individual rather than a group of individuals or diagnoses.
- The need to empower people by consulting and involving them in decisions about their own welfare and management.
- Recognising the validity of their perceptions about their ability to control their situation.

Social learning theory (observational learning)

Bandura et al. (1961) drew on the earlier learning theorists but examined how people can learn through observation of others to imitate some behaviours. This theory was later renamed as social cognitive theory.

Obviously we do not copy everyone all the time and it appears that some characteristics of models (people whom we may copy) make them more likely to be imitated. This includes people who we can see are:

- Similar to ourselves in some ways.
- Behave in role- or gender-appropriate ways.
- Have personal warmth.
- Are rewarded for their behaviour.
- Have power over resources.

Activity

When you are new to a job you may find that you are inclined to follow the example of a co-worker whom you have identified as showing good practice. Consider whether the co-worker may have some of these characteristics.

The knowledge that people have the ability to learn from others is used by parents, schools and workplaces where others are held up as good examples of desired behaviour. Examples include the public acknowledgement of achievements, introduction of student ambassadors and deliberate recruitment of people from under-represented groups into high-profile jobs. However, the role models that are copied may not necessarily be the ones that the organisation would choose. The class clown may well prove a more powerful model than the studious form captain.

Cases such as the murder of James Bulger, where it was suggested that the older boys were copying actors on violent videos, highlight some concerns about the extent that television and the media influence the way people act. This is far from clear cut, and is an important ongoing debate, but evidence suggests that it is unlikely to be a sole reason for extreme violent behaviour.

Developmental cognitive theory

Everyone is aware that children develop in their understanding and ability to solve problems. This is shown in the kind of tasks given to children, the way that they play and the expectation of how they explain events. You would not be surprised by a 5 year old talking about the toys coming alive and playing at night but you would not usually expect a 15 year old to hold the same beliefs.

Jean Piaget made a major contribution in stimulating studies on how children developed the ability to reason, understand and problem-solve. He suggested that this was related to their age and that learning opportunities needed to be appropriate for their stage of cognitive maturation. He emphasised that play and the opportunity to explore their environment were crucial in the development of children's cognitive ability.

Piaget identified that children pass through stages that typify their cognitive development, shown in Figure 7.2.

Sensori motor	0–2 years	Learning and understanding mainly through physical actions
Pre-operational	2–6 years	Using symbols such as words to represent objects Playing alongside other children A rather limited ability to understand others' position
Concrete	7–12 years	Capable of more complex thinking Beginning to understand rules of games and becoming capable of logical reasoning
Formal operations	12 onwards	Able to use abstract thinking, including thinking about themselves in more complex ways and identifying their personal morality

Figure 7.2 *Piaget's stages of cognitive development*

Piaget used the term 'schema' to explain how we adapt to our world through the way that we organise and build up knowledge. As we find out more about an object or event we take in or assimilate information. However, if the new information does not fit with our existing understanding it is necessary to alter our schema – a process called 'accommodation'. Driving this is the idea that we strive to be in *balance* or 'equilibrium', where new information becomes integrated into our schema, but *imbalance* stimulates us to seek more information. The ideal learning opportunities are considered to be when the imbalance is sufficiently stimulating and interests us in finding out more rather than too familiar or over-challenging.

Activity

Think about a time when you were given a task that really interested you and made you want to get on with it. Now try to recall times when the task just seemed too difficult so that you avoided it. Have you ever been bored at work because the job is not giving you sufficient challenge or interest?

Think of an example of how an understanding of the balance between 'known' and 'not known' could help you to devise learning activities for staff or clients.

Psychodynamic psychology

Sigmund Freud was the originator of this school but there have been other psychoanalytical psychologists after him who have adapted and developed these ideas.

Key points in Freud's ideas are that behaviour is assumed to be the result of unconscious process and previous experiences. The main drives or sources of motivation that govern human behaviour are described as the libido, associated with the sex drive and need to continue the species, and thanotos, the destructive force which is shown by aggression. He believed that the personality was formed from three parts: the id, ego and superego. Babies when they are born are dominated by their id (the pleasure principle). According to Freud they can only seek gratification to maintain their comfort, e.g. by crying when they are hungry or uncomfortable. As they get older they then start to develop the ego (the reality principle). This happens as they come to realise that they need to interact with people and the real world in order to get what they want. The final stage of personality development is through the acquisition of the superego. This acts as a conscience, which dictates what it is acceptable to want, with an accompanying sense of guilt if this is ignored.

The way that we view ourselves is so important to our well-being that Freud believed that we develop 'ego protective mechanisms'. Events or ideas that are potentially destructive to a positive view of the self are repressed from consciousness but remain within the unconscious and can affect behaviour many years later. Examples of ego defence mechanisms include denial: by suppressing awareness we can ignore painful or disturbing thoughts. When meeting clients you may be surprised that they did not seek advice and help about their debts or symptoms, even where they could indicate severe illness. Similarly those who are experiencing bereavement may not accept that someone has a terminal illness or has died.

According to early psychoanalytical theory, suppressing information was always harmful and therapy was needed to help people to recognise why they had suppressed these thoughts into their unconscious. However, it is now recognised that, at least in the short term, mechanisms such as denial can help in coming to terms with a severe and distressing problem.

Freud also believed that development went through a number of stages which were associated with areas of the body that provided a source of pleasure. If a child was not able to pass successfully through each stage then the child would be considered to be fixated and continue with typical behaviour into adulthood. For example, a person who drinks excessive alcohol could be assumed to have fixated at the oral stage or someone who is compulsively tidy fixated at the anal stage.

Erikson (1963) developed the psychoanalytical approach but suggested that development was characterised by conflict between the person's unconscious drives and their social world. Development of self-identity came as a result of resolving conflicts associated with eight life stages. These ranged from the first stage for the young baby of *trust versus mistrust* to the final stage of *integrity versus despair*.

Humanistic theories

These assume that individual development is through personal growth. Maslow (1970) proposed that everyone has an innate drive to achieve 'self-actualisation', which is a similar concept to that of realising our full potential. He suggested that this could only come about through essential needs being met and organised this into a 'hierarchy of needs' (Figure 7.3).

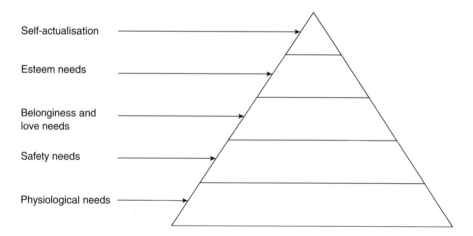

Figure 7.3 *Maslow's 'hierarchy of needs'*

You may feel that the idea of a hierarchy is too restrictive and there can be times when the need for that love or a need for respect can become more important than food or personal safety. However, it does emphasise that everyone has needs and that general well-being and development will be enhanced by their fulfilment.

The humanistic tradition underlies person-centred counselling based on the work of Carl Rogers which is further explored in Chapter 8.

Ecological theory

This theory is characterised by recognising the importance of individuals' whole environment (their ecosystem) when identifying influences on their development.

Bronfenbrenner (1979) identified this as being composed of:

- The microsystem – the immediate world of the individual, e.g. home, school and social activities.
- The mesosystem – the relationship between the various microsystems, e.g. home and school.
- The exosystem – the effect of wider influences, e.g. parents' working conditions and social activities.
- The macrosystem – the more indirect effects such as social institutions and ideologies, e.g. political decisions and the wider culture.

Associated with this theory is interest in how a child's personality and environment interact to lead the child to being 'at risk' of behavioural and developmental problems. Not all children seem to be equally vulnerable and Terrisse (2000) reviewed studies that identify factors that appear to be associated with risk or protection. These are seen as being significant at each level of the ecosystem so can include birth experience, socio-economic status, parental education and employment, school and recreational opportunities, government funding in supportive organisations and measures for providing equality of opportunities. Children who seem able to cope, despite experiencing some of these difficulties, are described as 'resilient'. It is through understanding what contributes to their ability to resist apparently adverse conditions that intervention programmes have been devised. These aim both to support and to modify the environmental stresses as well as promoting the development of the individual's own resources in coping. These approaches have been applied with a range of groups including aggression or drug taking in adolescence, children with disabilities, families in poor socio-economic conditions or those who have moved through immigration.

Although none of these theories is able to provide a complete explanation, together they help to build up our knowledge and gain understanding of the processes and influences on human behaviour. This is shown in the next section which looks at developmental psychology.

Lifespan development

Psychology is interested in not only recognising the changes that take place, but also identifying factors that might influence these changes.

Before reading further it would be helpful for you to reflect on your own life experiences and the factors that have influenced them.

Activity

The River of Life (how you came to be you)
Beginning with conception identify important landmarks in your life. This could include:

- o   Major life events: starting work, changes to relationships, illness, etc.
- o   Transitional life stages: adolescence, becoming a parent, ageing, etc.
- o   Transient life events: these could be very minor such as a conversation with someone at a crucial point in your life or seeing a television programme that affected your understanding of a social issue.

You might want to draw your own river of life and highlight key events/transitions. Try to think about what may have caused or influenced these changes.

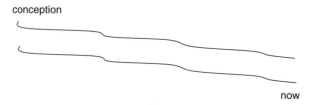

conception

now

In reflecting on your 'River of Life' you will have identified events that have personal significance as well as those that have similarities to others' experiences.

The areas of development that are being discussed in this section are:

- Two developmental processes:

    (a) The development of early social emotional relationships
    (b) The development of a self-concept.

- Two significant life periods:

    (a) Adolescence
    (b) Ageing.

Socio-emotional development of relationships

Relationships form a significant part in our lives and are important to development. You will be able to identify a number of your own significant relationships which could include parents, children, siblings, partners, work colleagues, friendship groups, care worker, clients and many others. Relationships may be important for different reasons and can be seen as essential to supporting and promoting development, as a source of satisfying our needs and for moderating stressful experiences. Those who are isolated and do not have close relationships can be some of the most vulnerable people in society.

It is assumed that there are behaviours that support or challenge the successful development of relationships and part of the explanation of how we acquire these skills is provided by studies of early social emotional development.

Video studies of new-born babies and their carers show how they engage in 'conversation' from soon after the baby is born and so start to establish their relationship. Babies are not passive dolls but participate and start to show their own needs, initiate and respond to the other person and communicate through sounds and eye gaze. Even very young babies show preferences for familiar people and can recognise smells and voices; they will look at faces with their complex shapes and movement rather than simpler patterns.

Shared time provides the opportunity for attachment between children and their carers. Bowlby (1969) described this as 'bonding' and proposed that the opportunity to develop specific attachments to others is an essential foundation for forming later relationships, including the ability to be sensitive and respond to the needs of others.

A child who has formed this attachment bond is assumed to show his or her attachment through behaviours including:

- Preference for the main carer.
- Greater willingness to be comforted by that carer.
- Using that carer as a safe base for exploring or returning to when feeling anxious.

What helps the development of these early relationships?

Clearly this must include some form of contact, but beyond this there are various parenting practices throughout the world with differences in attachment experiences and outcomes. Ainsworth et al. (1971) studied the responses of a child during a brief separation from the mother and suggested that the sensitivity and responsiveness of the parents would affect the child's security and confidence in forming later relationships. Some parenting classes will include sessions on facilitating new parents' understanding and responsiveness to their babies. However, while developing these interactional skills is important, it is necessary to recognise that individual differences in temperament, cultural practices and disabilities will also have an impact on early communication and its consequences.

THEORY BOX

Working just after the Second World War, **John Bowlby** studied the effect of separation between the mother and young child mainly within institutions. He described the consequences of separation from the mother as contributing to permanent long-term harm to the child's ability to develop relationships and integrate into society. From observations he described a child's responses to separation from the carer including:

- Protest: The child cries and shows anxiety about being separated.
- Despair: When this fails to bring about the return of the child's attachment figure, the child seems to be depressed, and becomes apathetic shown by reduced communication and play with others.
- Detachment: Following prolonged separation the child starts to form new attachments although these are mainly superficial and may be characterised by demonstrations of the child's uncertainty and loss of security in the predictability of new relationships.

However, Rutter (1972), while acknowledging potential harmful effects, also highlighted that the consequences would be affected by factors such as age, previous experience and how relationships were maintained during separation.

The demonstration of attachment behaviour between carer and child is considered one of the markers of a healthy relationship and is used by social workers and health professionals to inform their observations of quality of attachment experiences and responses to disruption and separation.

An important debate within our culture is the extent to which child and carer need to spend time together and the effect of separation through alternative care arrangements either as day care or longer periods. Some detrimental effects have been shown by group care of very young children; however, evidence also identifies the value of programmes that can enhance the different levels of the child's environment.

Any decision about the most appropriate childcare arrangements needs to consider:

- How the alternative care options can contribute to the child's development.
- Characteristics of the child including personal history, age and temperament.
- Sensitivity and quality of the day care provision.
- Relevance and support for the child's overall environment.

Applications of attachment theory are not limited to children. The consequences of disruption can be seen throughout life in experiences of grief and loss. This may occur through dissolution of peer or adult relationships or bereavement, loss of role from redundancy, or children leaving home. All have consequences for health and well-being.

This can help in understanding the way that people respond to problems such as a young child starting nursery school, the breakdown of a relationship or an older person entering a residential care setting. Attachment experiences influence how others respond to you which will affect the development of your self-concept.

Self-concept

The self-concept is defined as the way that we organise information into an understanding of what we think we are like. Psychologists often try to divide this understanding into different sections as it makes it easier to comprehend and study. This can include:

- An ideal self
- Body image
- Self-esteem.

The development of self-perception depends on increasing cognitive maturation in order to recognise, describe and eventually be able to reflect on the person that we have become. Learning about ourselves comes through the responses of others, their expectations, and the extent to which we meet them, as well as gaining self-knowledge through testing our own abilities.

During our development we incorporate the ideas of others into what we believe we should be like and so construct a self-ideal that may differ from our perception of what we are actually like. The bigger the difference between our ideal and our perceived reality, the more discontented and uncertain we may become. This personal evaluation is a measure of self-esteem.

This may involve self-questioning about:

- What we think we are worth.
- What we value about ourselves.
- What we tolerate as acceptable.
- What we like or despise about ourselves.

One of the aspects of ourselves that we can be particularly sensitive about is body image. The way that we think that we look can have an important effect on our behaviour and mood. If we believe that we look good, and fit somewhere near our ideal image, then we are more likely to feel comfortable and interact positively. Discontent with our image may severely affect our willingness to engage with others.

Body image includes the body size and shape, features, hair, smell, blemishes, colour and texture of skin. As part of ageing the body continues to change and there are particular points in people's lives when they have to come to terms with differences in their appearance. The onset of secondary sexual characteristics at adolescence coincides with an important stage in cognitive maturation. This stage allows individuals to think of themselves in more abstract terms so that they may be more self-conscious of their appearance and aware of how others might perceive them. It is also a period where there can be changes in social expectations as they look increasingly adult and sexually mature.

Other changes such as pregnancy, the early onset of baldness, changes in weight, disfigurement and ageing can all bring their own demands with a risk of negative re-evaluations and lowering of self-esteem. Increased self-awareness can lead to a fear of negative evaluation by others causing emotions such as embarrassment and shame.

Intervention programmes, aimed at helping people overcome their unhappiness or difficulties in fitting in with their social world, target self-esteem and use strategies to raise an individual's sense of self-worth and perception that others value the individual.

PRACTICE TIP

If we are to help clients cope with situations that may lead to embarrassment and shame it is essential to:

- Treat them as individuals and take time to understand their concerns and perceptions.
- Act in a professional and non-judgemental manner to help reassure them that otherwise socially taboo activities are acceptable in that therapeutic environment.
- Not show your own embarrassment or how the situation may be making you feel uncomfortable.

During development some periods assume particular significance. Some of the influences on development in childhood have already been discussed and the next section will consider the changes that are associated with adolescence and ageing.

Adolescence

Essentially this is the transitional period between childhood and adulthood and a time of considerable change that can make demands on the individual to adapt. Erikson (1963) considered this as a time of conflict between dependence and the need for autonomy progressing onto the stage of increasing need to develop a sense of self-identity.

Activity

Jot down the changes that you associate with adolescence and try to organise these into categories.

Some of the changes that you may have identified are:

- Physical changes including the adolescent growth spurt and the development of secondary sexual characteristics.
- Socio-emotional relationships with the increasing importance of peer groups and the development of adult sexual relationships.
- Increasing cognitive maturation increasing the ability to think in more abstract ways. This usually brings a greater capability for problem solving, reflection and independent decision making. It also often means more challenges to the self-concept and increasing self-consciousness.
- Social expectations and roles alter with age and increasing physical maturity. It is also a time when age or activities increase the likelihood of being stereotyped.

These changes are not necessarily going to develop at the same pace and can show wide variation between different people that may cause problems for the individual. Early sexual or physical maturity may occur before the cognitive development. Boys who experience late maturation tend to find themselves more isolated during their adolescence but more inclined to sensitivity and understanding in adulthood.

Despite general assumptions that adolescence is a difficult time, or that teenagers have problems, for many this is a period of development with successful adaptation to the changes. However, for others this will be a time of real concern with problems coming to the fore that may have long-term consequences.

At this point there is an increase in behavioural difficulties including conflicts at home and at school as well as a susceptibility to crime and antisocial activities. What is less clear is whether this is due to changes within the individual or social expectations. It is also a time often associated with the start of health-risk behaviours. Peer groups increase in significance in influencing behaviour as the teenager looks outside the family for a source of identity. When looking at the onset of adolescent smoking, Kobus (2003) pointed out that by behaving like others adolescents increase their acceptability to their peers. Belonging to a group provides a sense of belonging with opportunities for sharing social activities and the development of independence.

Another important time of transition comes with increasing age.

Ageing

Who is old?

There are many different ways of trying to decide when someone is old. Social policies will define retirement and pension age, cultural stereotypes vary over time and between societies, yet individuals have their personal understanding which may certainly change as they get older. People's perceptions will be influenced by their changing roles in society, health and fitness, comparison with others and personal expectations. Chronological age assumes less importance as people get older; this will be shown by widening differences in the ageing processes and emphasises the need to be aware of individuals' own view of their age.

Age a time of inevitable decline?

There is a common perception that old age is a time of inevitable decline and this is often reflected in the language that we use. However, for many older people there are positive benefits and it can be a very fulfilling period of their life.

Activity

Make a thought shower of the changes that you associate with ages.
   Try to group them under:

o Physical
o Cognitive
o Emotional
o Social

You may find that you need to add some other categories or that some things fit in more than one. Underline all the ones that seem to show the negative parts of growing older. If they are mostly negative, try to add others that may reflect more positive elements, such as greater confidence, acceptance of abilities or attributes, more leisure time and less demands being made on you.

Cognitive changes

Cognitive changes such as loss of memory, impaired problem solving or ability to undertake new learning are often a source of concern for people as they get older.

Some changes do take place, but this is more complex than assumptions that these can be measured by simply a loss of brain cells or is inevitable for a particular age group. These changes are not just about loss of function but also about the use of previously acquired skills, current situation and opportunities for mental activity and personal perceptions. It may be necessary to use different strategies to learn new information and activities can take more planning, but older people will be able to use their life experiences to help them achieve their objectives in spite of any reduction in speed of information processing. When working with older people it is essential to recognise that development varies in individuals and not to make assumptions based on ageist stereotypes.

Keeping physically and socially active does seem to contribute to successful ageing and maintaining health. This has been associated with the personality characteristics of hardiness which was identified by Kobasa (1979) and appears to aid in resisting stress and is linked to engaging in health protective behaviours (Magnani, 1990). Hardiness is characterised by a personal sense of control over their lives and events, commitment which implies involvement and interest and challenge, suggesting a willingness to engage and adapt to new experiences.

Bereavement and loss

These can occur at any age but will become increasingly likely with increasing age.

Bereavement can lead to a sense of loss regardless of the cause; it can arise from loss of a significant person, health, a home, even a lifestyle or pet. People can also suffer anticipatory grief, e.g. when someone is given a diagnosis of a fatal disease.

Russell (2000) identified the four main emotions associated with actual or anticipated loss as:

- Fear
- Anger
- Guilt
- Sadness.

Theorists such as Kübler-Ross (1969) suggest that there is a normal grieving process which requires the person to pass through specific stages of bereavement which may include periods of denial and depression, among others, before achieving acceptance.

For many people, bereavement is certainly associated with both physical and emotional consequences, which can increase mortality and the need for medical treatment. However, some help can contribute to moderating these harmful affects including:

- Social support
- Self-help groups
- Quality of care
- Being consulted and making decisions concerning the place of death.

Activity

Lifespan development
Identify how lifespan development theories and ideas can help in understanding behaviour associated with:

- o Childhood obesity
- o Adolescent smoking
- o An older person adjusting to moving into residential care.

The next section will consider further applications of psychology to working in the health and social care sector.

Psychology and working in health and social care

Stress

Stress usually results from a need to adapt to a changed situation and usually leads to an increase in physical arousal level.

THEORY BOX

The Yerkes–Dodson law (1908) explains the relationship between levels of arousal and when you are most effective in coping with the demands being made on you. It suggests that everyone has their individual optimal level of arousal where they perform best (Figure 7.4).

Too low a level of arousal leads to boredom and not using skills, but too high a demand brings about reduced ability to cope with the situation, increased inefficiency and potential for developing illness associated with stress.

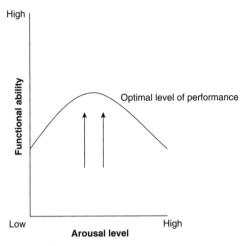

Figure 7.4   *The Yerkes–Dodson law – functional ability against arousal level*

Functional ability is how well you carry out your activities.

Arousal level is when there is an increase in physical and psychological responses to demands (how stressed you are).

Optimal level of performance is the level of arousal that allows you to work at your most efficient. Too low and you are probably bored; too high and you are unable to cope with the demands effectively.

C A S E   S T U D Y

Jason has been working as a supervisor on day duty within a supported housing setting for a number of years. Recently his partner left him and he is having difficulty arranging suitable access to his 7-year-old son. He is also finding himself in financial difficulties so has arranged to move to night duty for extra pay. Unfortunately he is having difficulties in sleeping. Managers are concerned that while he was previously very conscientious and meticulous they are finding work is being neglected and mistakes made. Some of the service users have complained that he has become angry, shouting at them with little provocation. A co-worker has mentioned his suspicions that Jason has started to drink very heavily.

As is demonstrated in the case study stress can have harmful effects including:

- Physiological:

    (a) short term, e.g. disruption, changes to appetite;
    (b) long term, e.g. increased risk of heart and vascular disease;
    (c) harmful changes to health behaviours, e.g. excessive drinking, smoking.

- Social and emotional:

    (a) aggression or apathy causing problems with relating to others;
    (b) unemployment and lowered income.

- Cognitive:

    (a) problem-solving abilities.

The transactional model of stress (Lazarus and Folkman, 1984)

This suggests that stress results from:

- A perception of the situation as threatening to our well-being.
- The perception of personal resources to be able to cope with the challenge.

A sense of stress may result from:

- The number of different and possibly competing challenges needing to be dealt with at the same time.
- A situation where previous methods of coping are either inappropriate or ineffective.
- There is insufficient social support.

It is important to recognise that a person's anxieties and responses are due to their interpretation of events and assumptions of their ability to cope, although these may appear trivial or unrealistic to others. Individuals will all respond differently to a breakdown in a relationship, moving schools, entering into a care home or adjusting to their own or someone else's illness.

Work within the health and social care field requires developing skills that help in managing personal and client's stressful experiences. This can include:

- Helping to develop more effective coping strategies, including looking at alternative ways of dealing with the problem or trying to change the negative emotions that have become linked to the situation.
- Using 'social support' from others through being given information or practical help, having someone show their belief in your ability to manage or just being part of a social network.

- Regaining a sense of control over the situations by facing the issues or starting to take actions that will eventually lead to possible solutions.

Changing health behaviour

It is now recognised that many of the modern illnesses and causes of death are related to people's lifestyle and behaviours. Diseases such as cardio-vascular disorders resulting in coronary artery disease, high blood pressure and strokes may be associated with diet, stress and lack of exercise. We are all familiar with health promotion campaigns that point out the health risks of cigarette smoking, drug taking or excessive drinking of alcohol. Other effects of behaviour on health are through whether we take part in screening programmes or to what extent we follow recommended treatments.

There are many situations in the health and social care field where help is needed to support people in changing or adopting behaviours to enhance the quality of their lives. This will include:

- Prompting or encouraging someone to seek advice from a health professional.
- Through an understanding of possible influences of changing behaviour, help in planning how to carry out changes.
- Providing support and understanding especially when they are having difficulties.
- Being ready to discuss treatment and rehabilitation programmes to make sure they understand the advice and can make informed choices.

Influences on health behaviours

Most people are aware that they could live a healthier lifestyle but for many an inability to change will lead to very real risks to their health. Influences involved in supporting and maintaining changes to health behaviours have been incorporated into theoretical models such as the health belief model (Becker and Rosenstock, 1984).

THEORY BOX

The health belief model suggests that whether we take action, i.e. change our behaviour, is influenced by:

- **Individual variables:** This includes things like our age, sex, religious beliefs, knowledge and experiences of ourselves or friends and family.

(Continued)

> *(Continued)*
>
> - **Perceived vulnerability:** These variables can affect how seriously we consider the consequences of not taking action as well as to what extent we consider ourselves to be at risk.
> - **Cost and benefits:** Part of deciding whether to take action will be based on an assessment of perceived benefits compared with anticipated costs. Costs can include financial over such as joining a gym but would also include time, increased anxiety or embarrassment.
> - **Cues to action:** Check-up reminders, media articles or contact with someone who has become ill can all act as prompts to take action.

Other influences on whether we act more healthily include:

- **Attitudes:** The theory of reasoned action suggests that forming an intention to change health behaviours will be determined both by our own attitudes towards a particular behaviour and by an awareness of other people's attitudes. This can be seen when children or adolescents start to smoke, because that is considered to be the right way to behave by other members of their group, or in decisions about breast feeding being influenced by partners' or parents' attitudes.
- **Reinforcement:** Operant conditioning identified how we are more likely to carry out behaviour that is reinforced. A behavioural change plan should be designed to have clear achievable steps that can be reinforced by acknowledgement of success, such as praise or treats, provided either by others or ourselves.
- **Self-efficacy beliefs:** Self-efficacy refers to our belief about whether we can succeed in making changes. If we have a high self-efficacy we will have greater expectations and confidence in our ability to change. Working with service users can involve both assessing their self-efficacy beliefs and introducing strategies to increase them.

A related idea is outcome expectancies. Again you are more likely to attempt to change your behaviour if you believe the effort will bring about the outcome that you actually want.

Activity

Decide on a behaviour that you believe would make you healthier. Examples might be drinking more water, giving up chocolate, reorganising your life/work balance or changing your diet to include more vegetables.

Try to change this behaviour for a week and keep a diary of the type of things that helped or made it more difficult. Find examples from the influences that have been discussed in this section.

Carrying out this activity can help highlight the problems people encounter when changing health behaviours.

Observation and report writing

Observation and making reports is an integral part of most care work, yet as everyone is aware it is possible to make mistakes through not noticing all the relevant information, forgetting or misinterpreting what we have seen.

Part of this is due to our attempts to make sense of the world. Information about our environment comes through the senses: sight, smell, sound, taste and touch. However, our ability to take notice of these stimuli is selective. Perception is the way that we select, process, interpret and draw inferences about the meaning of the information that we have received. This will be influenced by previous experiences, learning and personal significance.

Through experience we develop our personal schemas and understanding of the world which influence what we notice and can predict how we respond. Schema represents our reality rather than a true reflection of the actual world and is unique to the individual.

Our schemas lead us to take more notice of the familiar and information that supports our existing ideas. The result is that we can miss unexpected symptoms or behaviours that do not fit in with our expectations.

Activity

Since working on and studying psychological aspects relevant to health and social care issues, consider how you have become more aware of related topics in the media.

Reflect upon your developing awareness of the psychological needs of service users.

How do you think you have become more aware of people's emotional and social needs?

Stereotyping

Through our perceptions we simplify and organise information that contributes to the formation of stereotypes. This tendency to over-generalise from very limited information is a characteristic of human behaviour. It does have important implications when working in the health and care sector. Challenging the tendency to use stereotypes and generalisations helps the care professional to focus on the needs of the individual rather than provide care that is based on the assumed needs of 'the elderly, nursery-age children or people with learning difficulties'.

Some terms are particularly powerful, especially where they have negative connotations. A report on a new service user that included words such as 'difficult, demanding, aggressive or manipulative' could affect how staff approach the person and influence perceptions of their behaviour.

Attribution theory

We not only observe people, but also make judgements about the causes of their behaviour. Actions are often attributed to being the result of either personality characteristics of the person or recognition of how they have been influenced by the situation. These cognitive biases make us more ready to see our own behaviours resulting from the situation that we are in, while seeing other's behaviour as mainly determined by their personality characteristics. An example would be:

> I failed the exam because I was so busy at work; they failed the exam because they are too lazy to study.

The following tips will be helpful when writing reports or passing on information.

PRACTICE TIPS

Be aware of the need to:

- Be objective rather than subjective. When reporting on an individual talk about your actual observations not assumptions about the individual's character.
- Avoid stereotypical and judgemental language.
- Make use of care plans to identify how to meet the needs of an individual rather than assumptions based on group membership.
- Keep an open mind. If someone has a specific condition, still take notice of other symptoms or behaviours.
- Make judgements about the reasons for behaviour. Think about how the situation could contribute to people's actions.
- Use the organisational records to make sure that you are not ignoring relevant information.
- Write down information as soon as possible to make sure that you are accurate.

SUMMARY

Psychology seeks to understand and explain the causes and consequences of behaviour.

The different psychological theories all contribute to an understanding of the influences on human behaviour.

It is necessary to recognise the complexity of behaviour and that observed behaviour is affected by cognitions, emotions, physiological status and social interactions.

The study of psychology can enhance delivery of care through greater understanding of service users' behaviour, how to support them in meeting their needs and promoting their well-being. It will also help in reaffirming the importance of treating people as individuals and increasing awareness of potential factors that can challenge our objectivity in planning and delivering care.

Awareness of psychological processes contributes to personal and professional development including management of issues such as stress and health protective behaviour.

Further reading

This chapter has introduced a range of psychological issues that are relevant to your work in health and social care. In order to develop your studies further, aim to find additional readings and books that fit with your existing knowledge level but provide additional detail, different perspectives or applications.

There are many very good psychology texts; some will provide a general approach while others will cover a specific area, subdivision of psychology or practice focus. This list includes a few to help direct your further reading.

Russell, G. (2000) *Essential psychology for nurses and other health professionals*. London. Routledge. A very readable text; although some of the examples are based in clinical settings most are applicable to the wider health and care sector.

Crawford, K. and Walker, J. (2003) *Social Work and Human Development*. Exeter, Learning Matters. Provides an overview with useful case studies and learning activities to reinforce your understanding. Although directed at social work, the emphasis on practice can be applied to a wider area of health and social care work.

Smith, P., Cowie, H. and Blades, M. (2002) *Understanding Children's Development*, 4th edn. Oxford: Blackwell. A comprehensive text that will provide the opportunity for further study of development in children.

Walker. J., Payne, S., Smith, P. and Jarrett, N. (2004) *Psychology for Nurses and the Caring Professions*, 2nd edn. Maidenhead: Open University Press. Case studies and questions make this a useful book for exploring some of the issues raised in this chapter in more detail.

Albery, I., Chandler, C., Field, A., Jones, D., Messer, D., Moore, S., Stirling, C. and Davey, G. (2004) *Complete Psychology*. London: Hodder and Stoughton. An extensive introduction into general psychology which could serve as a valuable resource for developing further reading and understanding.

8 INTERPERSONAL COMMUNICATION

Judith Mann

SUMMARY CHAPTER CONTENTS

- Your role as a care worker
- Communication skills
- The structure of interaction
- Working in groups
- Barriers to communication
- Managing conflict situations
- Summary

Learning objectives

By the end of this chapter, you should be able to:

- Understand the importance of effective communication.

- Recognise a range of communication skills.

- Monitor and evaluate your use of communication skills.

- Gain knowledge about groups and group behaviour.

- Reflect on 'difference' within the communication process.

- Recognise barriers to communication.

- Learn how to manage conflict situations.

Introduction

You have made a choice to pursue a career in health and social care, working with people who, at the particular time at which you are involved with them, will be feeling 'vulnerable'. The skills that you will need will primarily be those which many of us take for granted, but which you will need to develop in order to enhance work with the service user, and if appropriate the carer.

Effective communication skills underpin all the values which you, as a health and social care worker, need in your work with people. These are the skills by which people judge you. Your development of these skills and the way that you interact with people will be reflected in the work that you do. The skills are important in your day-to-day contact with people who may require your help and support. They are important when you meet prospective service users for the first time, in maintaining an ongoing relationship or in the assessment and review process.

Your values and moral principles (which are explored in Chapter 5), and how you convey them, are what help to make you a professional care worker. They ensure that you consider the needs of the service user and keep them central to your interactions with people. A failure to achieve this can result in the service user losing confidence in you as a worker, a factor that can greatly impede and disadvantage ongoing work.

This chapter will provide you with relevant knowledge which will enable you to reflect on your communication skills and appreciate their importance when working with people.

Your role as a care worker

Partnership working

The National Health Service and Community Care Act 1990 emphasises the importance of working with service users and carers in a way that ensures that their views are listened to and that their choices are considered. The care worker's role in health and social care is centred on the needs of a vulnerable person – child or adult. This involves the worker being able to be aware of that person as an individual with whom they are 'in partnership' in their care.

> A vulnerable person is someone who is in need of community care services by reason of mental, age or any other disability and 'who may be unable to take care of him or herself' (DoH, 2000: 8–9).

New Labour's modernising agenda for Public Services (1998) emphasised the importance of 'a partnership approach throughout the whole system of public services'. This means not only the services working together, but the professionals and service users working with each other in this way.

One way in which you approach this notion of partnership will be evidenced by your use of effective communication skills. Your use of these skills will convey to the service users your attitude towards them and how you intend to work with them. For example, a community care assistant will often be required to assist an older person in the task of dressing. In taking the service user's views into consideration, the community care assistant would ask the person what they would like to wear that day and how much assistance they require with dressing. This action demonstrates making decisions *with* people, not *for* people.

The following activity will help you to consider further requirements of an effective helping role.

Professional approach

Activity

Think of a situation in which you need to go to someone for help: for example, an interview with your GP about a problem or symptom that has been worrying you for sometime; a discussion with a health visitor about the feeding pattern of your newly born baby; a discussion with a tutor at college about writing an essay on a subject you are studying.

o   What did you expect from the professional?
o   How did the professional respond to you?

You would most likely want the professional to take your concerns seriously by listening to you. You would also want something from the professional: advice, reassurance or acceptance of your concerns. What would be most important would be that you were listened to and that you felt valued as a person.

We all appreciate being treated as individuals; none of us likes to be treated as a category, e.g. 'old person', 'youth', 'disabled', 'resident'. In care work the way we address people, and the way that we speak about them and to them, are significant in demonstrating our respect for the people that we care for and work with.

> The professional worker should respond to you as a 'person', not to you as a 'category', i.e. *patient, new mother, parent, student*. The Valuing People White Paper (DoH, 2001), although specifically directed at people with learning disabilities sets the standard for services to respond to individual need.

In the activity above, the professional that you saw needed to demonstrate a range of qualities and characteristics in order to give you that sense of being attended to as a *person*. What do you think these qualities were able to do?

- Did they make you feel that you mattered?
- Do you think the professional responded to you with interest?
- Was the professional attentive to your needs?
- Was the focus of the interaction on you?

Such characteristics and qualities could be described as empathy, having a non-judgemental approach, and demonstrating respect for you as an individual.

Person-centred care

Putting the person at the centre of the interaction is not a new concept. Carl Rogers, the distinguished American counsellor and psychotherapist, spent most of his life refining an approach he called the person-centred approach. He emphasised that it was the attitude of the worker, in his case, the counsellor towards the client, that gave it its *person-centredness* or *client-centredness*. The helper should demonstrate *empathy, genuineness*, and *respect* as the *core conditions* of the helping relationship. If the counsellor offered these and used effective communication skills, then a feeling of helping would follow.

Rogers' core conditions can be applied to all helping roles and in particular to care work. Consider what is meant by the word *empathy*. You may be more familiar with the notion of *sympathy*. Sympathy is when someone is sorry for you. This can be helpful in the first instance, but it does not necessarily help you to resolve your problem. However, empathy is when someone demonstrates an understanding of your situation *as you are experiencing it, is respectful of your point of view* – not judging you or discriminating against you and giving you the feeling that they were *genuinely* there to help you. Their words match their feelings (Rogers, 1951). Empathy is to feel *with*, sympathy is to feel *like* (Stewart, 1992).

To demonstrate that you have empathy with service users is to understand their position, recognise their condition and respect their point of view. Rogers (1951) described empathy as the ability to 'sense the client's world as if it were your own'.

Characteristics of a helper

Your role as a care worker is different from that of a counsellor, but there are many similarities in the characteristics of all helping roles. To be an effective helper it is generally recognised that these qualities should be demonstrated, qualities and characteristics such as:

- Empathy and being non-judgemental.
- Being genuine.
- Showing respect for the person.
- Being non-discriminatory and honest.
- Having good listening skills.
- Demonstrating warmth towards the person.
- Being likable.
- Adopting a professional approach.
- Being a good communicator.
- Being aware of the need for confidentiality.

These characteristics are skills that can also be learned; they are characteristics that your service users will want you to evidence. Taken together they will enable you to demonstrate effective communication skills which become essential for your relationship with the people you work with.

Self-management and self-presentation

Care work involves your 'self' more than some other forms of work. As a care worker you need to consider how you relate to the other people you meet during your working day, most especially service users and carers. This involves how much information you may reveal about yourself and how you present your self to others.

This information you reveal about yourself to others is referred to as 'self-disclosure'. It becomes important in helping relationships as Myers and Myers (cited in Burton and Dimbleby, 1988) state:

> A relationship develops only when you and the other person are willing to go through the mutual process of revealing yourself to each other. If you can't reveal yourself, you cannot be close. To be silent about yourself is to be a stranger. (Burton and Dimbleby, 1988: 33)

Johari's window (Luft and Ingham, 1969, cited in Hartley, 1993) illustrates different types of information about the 'self' and shows how the 'self' changes through interaction.

The window has four 'panes'(Figure 8.1). Each 'pane' represents information about the 'self'. You can experiment by putting your own information into the different 'panes'. Consider how you feel about the different information, how readily you might reveal it and to whom:

- **Public pane:** This is information most people would willingly share: what job they do, how they would describe themselves, which town they live in; the answer to the question 'Who am I?'
- **Private pane:** This is information that is personal and private to yourself which you would not so easily share with others: your medical history, your family background, the contents of your bank account.

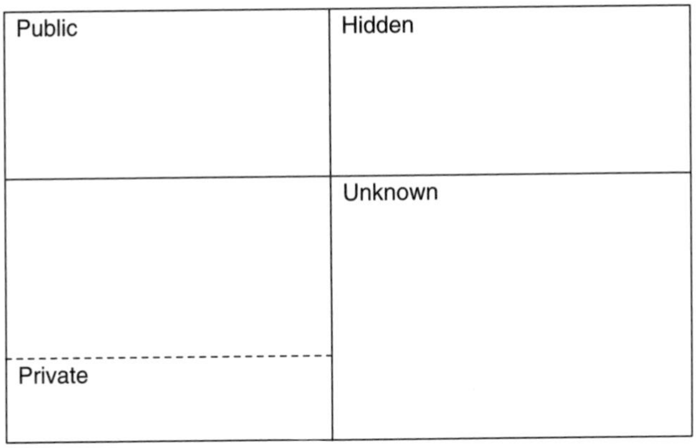

Public	Hidden
	Unknown
Private	

Figure 8.1   *Johari's window*

- **Hidden pane:** Information known to other people that is not known to you. How others see you, your bad habits or the special qualities that you are unaware of.
- **Unknown pane:** This represents your potential: what you might be capable of through personal and professional development; where you might be when you finish your course of study.

Johari's window is a useful way to consider how you relate to other people. The key way to make successful relationships within or outside work is to reveal information *appropriately* about yourself. It is important to think about this when developing a professional approach with service users. They will want to tell you about themselves as well as listen to you. The 'window' demonstrates a useful model for when information is shared appropriately; the person's 'private pane' increases as they extend their 'public pane' (see the dashed line in Figure 8.1). In sharing yourself with others you will discover more about both them and yourself. In order to do this you need to communicate effectively.

Self-presentation

As well as being aware of how much you reveal to service users, as a care worker you need to give consideration as to how you present yourself in the working environment and to service users and the impact this may have. This will be particularly important in the work-based learning element of your Foundation Degree.

Self-presentation consists of the manner and attitude which you put forward, and also aspects of your appearance. Self-presentation becomes an aspect of non-verbal communication – you are communicating something about yourself. Your dress, hair, make-up, jewellery, any piercings, and visible tattoos all say something about who you are and about yourself.

Some employers will have strong views on how you should present yourselves for work; some of these will be based on health and safety. They will not want you to put yourself or the service users at unnecessary risk. You may be required to wear a uniform and may want you to remove jewellery and piercings while at work. Most importantly they will want you to be neat, clean and tidy. These aspects will also be important to consider when you attend for interview.

When you give consideration to the above components of non-verbal communication, you are conveying a professional approach to your work.

Communication skills

Communication skills can be divided into written, verbal and non-verbal communication. Written communication is vital for accurate record keeping and is likely to involve information about the care needs of service users such as care plans, handovers, assessments and other reports. Information that is written down in this way should contain factual information that is objective, valid and reliable. It should inform rather than direct action.

This chapter is mainly concerned with 'interpersonal communication': that is, *communication between persons* which is verbal and non-verbal. Non-verbal communication is communication which does not involve words, such as facial expression, but which conveys much meaning.

The skills of interpersonal communication

An interpersonal skill is *any skill which is part of interpersonal communication and which can be learned, practised and improved upon.* The person sending the message and the person receiving the message are subject to a number of social, environmental and psychological influences.

There are a range of interpersonal skills that you will need to be aware of. These include:

- Empathy.
- Self-presentation.
- Being aware of and using non-verbal communication.
- Listening.
- Questioning.
- Establishing rapport.
- Attending.
- Using touch and personal space.

- Observing.
- Clarifying.
- Reflecting.
- Summarising.
- Being able to conclude and end an interaction.

Listening

Until you think about it carefully many people would not regard listening as a skill. Listening is something that they do (or do not do) without thinking about it!

Consider what is involved in listening. When you are next with a friend, or with a child, make a point of paying closer attention to what they are communicating, not just the words they use but their facial expressions. This should involve your full attention. To give your full attention to someone else is hard work because you have to concentrate!

Think about how you listen to people most of the time. Most people only really listen to a percentage of what they hear. They are selective listeners and tune in and out of the conversation unless it is something in which they are particularly interested.

Being a good listener is about:

- Giving your full attention.
- Maintaining eye contact.
- Following the story.
- Sitting or standing near to the speaker at a reasonable distance.
- Looking interested in what people have to say.
- Interrupting them as little as possible.
- Making appropriate comments to them indicating that you are responding to what they have to say.

One of the key skills which you will be demonstrating is that of *attending*, demonstrating by your *non-verbal communication* that you are interested in what they have to say.

Attending

Attending involves:

- Sitting squarely and facing the person at a slight angle.   (S)
- Having an open posture.   (O)
- Leaning slightly to show interest.   (L)
- Giving eye contact.   (E)
- Having a relaxed posture.   (R)

The acronym SOLER should help you to remember the skill of *attending*.

Practise this skill the next time you are required to listen to what someone has to say and see what difference it makes to them. If possible ask them if it made a difference. If you use this skill effectively you will have demonstrated that you were an *active listener* and that the speaker will know by your non-verbal communication that you have heard and understood what they had to say.

The structure of interaction

An interaction describes *action* between persons. This is generally referred to as face-to-face communication. It is only one aspect of communication as communication can take other forms, namely written, verbal, non-verbal, electronic.

Interaction is interpersonal, literally between people, and can be one to one or in a group with two or more people.

Structure refers to the process of interaction. An interaction can be formal, such as an interview, or informal, such as a casual chat, but still has a beginning, a middle and an end. Nelson-Jones (1997) refers to the first part of this process as 'meeting, greeting and seating'. It may or may not have a purpose, such as a job interview, it may simply be social, but this also has an outcome.

As a health and social care worker your interactions can influence the other person's sense of well-being. This requires you to think more carefully about how you communicate with your service users.

Just ask yourself when you are next in a working or college environment:

- How often do you plan what you want to say?
- Do you think about how you should say things?
- How often do you get distracted in the middle of a conversation?
- Have you ever been so distracted that you leave the person you have been talking to without finishing the conversation, perhaps leaving the other person feeling uncared for and not listened to?

Think about the structure of an interaction.

Activity

Thinking about the structure of an interaction

Watch a couple of interviews on television and observe the interaction:

○ Did the interview have a structure?
○ Could you recognise:

   (a) A beginning
   (b) A middle
   (c) An ending?

- o What actions or activities did the interviewer demonstrate to give the interview its structure in each section?
- o What skills of interpersonal communication did the interviewer demonstrate?
- o Can you identify any other skills which the interviewer used?

The beginning should have a greeting, preferably using the person's preferred form of address. This should have helped put the person at their ease.

The middle should show that the interviewer was able to demonstrate good listening skills, perhaps adopting 'SOLER'. The interviewer may have shown empathy and listened to any concerns of the interviewee.

At the end the conversation should be concluded and closed, perhaps with a thank you and goodbye.

Now that you have thought about the structure of an interaction, think back to the examples you were asked to think about in the first activity, when you wanted to be treated as an individual, and relate this to a health and social care environment.

Non-verbal communication

Non-verbal communication is that type of communication which happens *without* words. In the second activity, it was suggested that you watch interviews on television to study the structure of an interaction. This activity can also be useful in studying non-verbal communication.

Activity

Watch an interview on television by turning down the sound and only watching the movements that people make.

Write down what you notice about the two people and the way they interact. This will encourage you to focus on non–verbal communication. You will notice that you become a much better observer of behaviour.

Did you manage to observe some of the following components of non-verbal communication? They are sometimes referred to as *paralanguage*:

- **Spatial distance and personal space** – how far apart each person sits and how they use the space between them.
- **Touch** – whether or not there is any physical contact between them.
- **Head movements** – nods, shakes and inclinations of the head.
- **Body movements** – movements of the whole body.

- **Leg and foot movements** – crossed/uncrossed legs.
- **Gestures** – movements of the hands and arms.
- **Facial expressions** – smiles and other movements of the face.
- **Dress, jewellery, hair, make-up** – adornments of the body, which are part of self-presentation.
- **Posture and orientation** – the way a person is standing/sitting and the way one person is angled towards another person.
- **Voice** – volume (how much they speak), tone, pitch, intonation (the ups and downs of speech), rate (how fast they speak). These components of non-verbal communication (*NVCs*) are to do with voice or speech rather than words and are therefore also part of non-verbal communication. By turning up the television and listening to the voices of the interviewer and interviewee, you will be able to hear some of the emotion conveyed in what they are saying.

It is worth considering a couple of areas of non-verbal communication a bit further as they seem to be particularly relevant in health and social care.

Spatial distance and personal space are important areas because, when working with people, you may be entering their own personal space at home. Personal space (proximity or territory) refers to that space around a person which feels part of themselves.

Activity

Next time you are in a classroom at college, note how you and your fellow students manage your personal space:

- ○ Do you sit it your usual place in the classroom and then regard it as your chair?
- ○ Experiment with moving around the room yourself and sitting in different places.
- ○ How does it feel to sit in a different place?

Personal space for service users may be apparent in that they may have their favourite chair to sit in. People may want their possessions kept in a particular place. You will need to respect their personal space and talk to them about what you need to do to help them. You will need to ask permission to provide the care they need and perhaps be entering into the different zones of a person's space.

Hall (1966) identified that individuals have different zones around them which suit different situations:

- Your 'intimate' zone is a distance around you of up to 18 inches (45 cm). Your intimate zone is normally entered only by family, friends, children, partner, close friends and pets!

- Your 'personal' zone is a distance of 1½–4 feet (0.5–1.2 m) and is normally entered by acquaintances and people that you know fairly well.
- The 'social' zone is a distance of 4–12 feet (1.2–3.7 m) and entered by other friends and acquaintances, work colleagues.
- A 'business' zone, which is regarded as a distance of 12–20 feet (3.7–6 m), would be for those people you know less well at formal meetings and through business.
- While a person's public' zone of about 20 feet (6 m) or more would be for strangers or people you know less well.

Observation of these zones is very important in a social interaction.

It is also important when thinking about 'personal space' or 'territory' that you recognise cultural and individual differences. Some people that you work with – both work colleagues and service users – may represent this variation. Some will 'invade' your territory, and some will feel 'invaded' by your approaching them at what you consider to be a 'safe' distance. This is especially true when working with people with an impairment – hearing, or learning disability, or dementia – where there may be a difficulty in 'reading' non-verbal communication.

PRACTICE TIPS

- Develop your own sensitivity to non-verbal communication (NVCs).
- Be observant to the needs of others.
- Make sure that you get to know the people/service users you are working with.
- Communicate with people as you approach them.
- Approach people from a face-to-face orientation, rather than from where they cannot see you.
- Take advice from other care workers.

Your skills of observation will be very important in recognising non-verbal communication. Observation may not just involve 'seeing' but also involve using other 'senses' of smell, hearing, touch if appropriate and perhaps what might be called a 'sixth sense', one of intuition, where you sense all is not well with the other person.

Touch

As a care worker whose role may be to provide personal care to a vulnerable person, you may assume that it is appropriate for you to 'invade someone's space' in order to provide this care. However, you will now recognise from considering the zones associated with personal space that this has to be managed very carefully. It is important that boundaries of touch are carefully observed. Communication skills can help you achieve your working goals in the most person-centred way, by maintaining respect and dignity towards those for whom you provide care.

Activity

Think of three ways in which you can use these skills to maintain the dignity of a disabled person when giving assistance with personal care.

1

2

3

As a community care worker these might involve:

1 When assisting someone with bathing, using a towel as much as possible to maintain dignity and privacy.
2 Finding out how much assistance they might need with dressing.
3 Promoting choice in decisions about what to wear.

Questioning skills

Most people would not think of 'questioning' as a skill of interpersonal communication. However, questions are the way that we find out about people and are fundamental to how we make relationships.

A question is the first greeting when people meet each other: **How are you?**

Questions can be divided into two main types – 'open' questions and 'closed' questions.

'How are you?' is an open question, because it can be answered in many different ways. A closed question is one that allows only a one-word or yes/no response. For example:

• 'What day is it today?'
• 'Would you like to wear these black trousers?'
• 'Shall I make you some toast?'

Most questions begin with one of the following: what, where, which, when, why and how? A quick way of referring to these is as the *5WH*. This is not the only way a sentence may be made into a question, but it is a frequent method.

Closed questions are frequently used to find out facts. They can be useful in quickly making an assessment of a situation and obtaining a history or the person's background.

Think how you might change the following questions into more 'open' questions:

'Have you eaten breakfast today?'.................... 'Yes'

'Would you like a bath?'..................................... 'No'

'Which socks would you like to wear?'............ 'The blue ones'

Open questions give a person the opportunity to respond in a variety of ways:

'What would you like for breakfast?' .... 'I'd like some porridge followed by some toast'

What would you like to wear today?' .... 'I'd like to wear my white shirt, black trousers and my blue socks'

Generally you will find out more about someone, or their situation, by asking open questions.

Questions can also be framed by: Altering your tone of voice, by raising it at the end of a sentence:

'You'd like to wear your blue socks?'

Or responding in what is called a 'reflective' way:

'Did you say you wanted to wear your blue socks?'

This tells the person that you have listened to them and that what you heard was correct. This is called *clarifying*.

Not all questions are helpful. The use of the word 'why' at the beginning of a sentence can be rather intimidating:

'Why are you wearing your blue socks?'

('Oh dear, my others are dirty!')

Try getting someone to ask you some 'why' questions about what you are wearing and see how it feels.

Questions, when well used, can be a great way of developing good working relationships.

Reflecting and paraphrasing

These are skills of interpersonal communication which assist with the listening and clarifying aspects of an interaction.

Reflecting can be used to ask a question as mentioned above, or it can be used to demonstrate your attention to what someone has said. Reflecting can have two aspects: reflection of content or reflection of feeling.

Reflection of content

Reflection of content can also be called paraphrasing, but there is a slight difference between the two. Reflection of content is when it is primarily the speaker's words that are reflected back to the speaker. Paraphrasing is when the content of the speech is reflected back in the listener's words but in a way that captures the meaning. It can be a useful way of summarising what the person has said.

Hartley (1993: 46) refers to the use of key words as a way of encouraging the speaker to say more about a particular subject. This is helpful when a counsellor or other helper wants to encourage someone to 'elaborate'. For example:

Statement: I have always wanted to travel to Kenya.

Question: *To Kenya?*

Response: Yes, ever since I watched 'Born Free' as a child.

Reflection of feeling

As has been mentioned above, non-verbal communication often conveys what people feel about a subject they are talking about. This can be conveyed by tone of voice, facial expression or body movement or gesture. A skilled observer will notice that there is feeling behind the words spoken.

The following is a variation on the conversation above:

Statement: I had a plane ticket booked and then my mother became ill and I had to cancel it. It was all right, though, because I knew I would go later on.

Response: You sound a bit regretful that you got as far as booking your flight and then were unable to make the journey.

Statement: Well, yes, it did feel like a missed opportunity.

Using reflection enables one person to discover much more about the other person's underlying emotion.

The above skills are important in demonstrating *empathy* in communication.

Concluding and ending

This section began by looking at the structure of interactions. There are friendly ways of greeting people – for example, smiling, saying 'hello', and using their name. These are very good ways of 'getting off on the right foot'.

It is also important to end your interaction in a positive way. This might involve saying when you will see the person again, confirming any future arrangements and saying 'goodbye'. This is the skill of concluding/ending.

Any interaction will have a conclusion or an ending, which should leave both parties feeling satisfied with what has taken place and that a reasonable outcome has been achieved.

The conclusion might involve one person summarising what has taken place. It might involve arrangements for the next meeting with a clarification of the time and place. It will most certainly involve social factors such as saying goodbye, and some sort of pleasantries about what has taken place – if that is appropriate.

Working in groups

Communication within groups is more complicated than communication on a one-to-one basis. Most health and social care workers will work in teams, even if they interact with service users on a one-to-one basis. They will need effectively to pass on information and learn to work with different co-workers.

When thinking about working in a group it is important to think about membership of the group. Most people will want to feel that they are a part of that group or team to which they belong.

Activity

Think of social groups to which you belong.

What makes you feel part of that group? Is the group composed of like-minded people? What do you have in common?

A working group usually has a goal or purpose in common, but it might not work effectively. Working effectively usually requires more than a common goal.

Groups have different sets of needs which are referred to as:

- Task
- Maintenance
- Individual needs

as in Figure 8.2.

Task needs are those to do with the task or purpose for which the group has been set up. This might be the *aim* of the group or *mission statement* of the company. It is the reason why the group or team has been brought together. The task needs of a group would be to do with 'getting the job done'. This is the more formal aspect of group life.

Maintenance or social needs of a group are to do with what makes being part of a group enjoyable – it is the fun side of group life. It is getting together at a Christmas party or going out for a drink after work. It is having a chat over a cup of coffee or finding out that your children are at the same school.

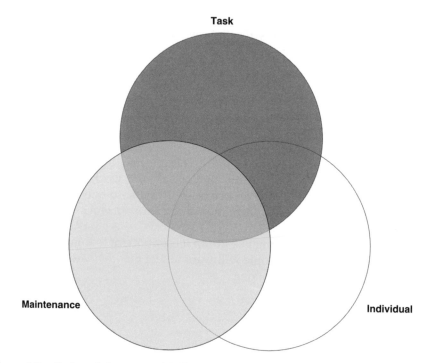

Task

Maintenance

Individual

Figure 8.2   Task, maintenance and individual needs in groups

Individual needs are the needs of each individual group member. They are the personal aspects we bring to the group – our own attitudes, skills and values – our own individual 'agenda'. To some extent these are superseded by the needs of the group as a whole, but they cannot be ignored.

There is an overlap between these sets of needs which makes every group unique.

If a group were concerned solely with the task needs it would be a very formal group. If the group were concerned only with the social or maintenance aspect, it would never get any work done! If each individual were concerned only with their own needs, the group would not work towards its common goal!

So what, therefore, makes for an effective group?

An effective group is likely to have the following characteristics:

- A common goal
- Two-way communication
- Leadership that is democratic

- A sense of group cohesion
- Conflict that is seen as positive
- High-problem-solving capacity. (Johnson and Johnson, 1998)

Activity

Consider which of the groups you belong to are 'effective' groups.

There are, of course, different types of groups. Tajfel and Fraser (1978) have suggested the following:

- Family groups
- Friendship groups
- Work groups.

Each of these groups has been set up for a different purpose. Each will have a different set of *norms* or behaviours which are associated with being a member of that group. Knowing the norms of a group gives you a better chance of acceptance into that group. Of course you may not always want to conform to the norms of a particular group, but that will depend on your own value base.

The 'life' of a group

Some groups are set up for a specific purpose and only last for a particular period of time. One aspect of groups is that they change over time – they go through a process of evolution. Tuckman's model (cited in Inskipp, 1996) provides a framework for tracking the changes in a group over time. His stages are:

- **Forming:** This stage is when a group first meets together. The task may be set, but the way to achieve it may be unclear. Group members are uncertain of each other and their own roles. They worry about belonging to the new group and whether other members will accept them.
- **Storming:** This next stage is when the group members are more familiar with each other and may jockey for position within the group. There may be conflict between group members as they negotiate the task and there may be competition for leadership.
- **Norming:** The group members begin to settle down with each other. Group roles begin to be established. There is an open exchange of views and a friendly atmosphere develops.
- **Performing:** This is the most productive stage of group life. There is a good sense of group cohesion. Members pull together and they work together to carry out the task.

- **Mourning:** The natural span of the group has come to an end. The task will have been achieved or the reason fulfilled its purpose. The group members begin to disband. There is talk of a reunion and an ending has been achieved.

Not all groups will go through all of these stages and they may get 'stuck' at one stage and not move beyond it. This will depend upon how effective the group is and on the group's problem-solving capacity. You may not always be aware of the stages a group has gone through, because it depends when you joined that group. Unless you were there at the beginning it will have a history that preceded your membership.

Roles in groups

This relates to the different individuals in a group and the roles they play. As Shakespeare wrote in *As You Like It*:

All the world's a stage,
And all the men and women merely players.

We perform roles in a variety of situations: we do not just have work roles such as care workers, but we have social roles, professional roles, family roles, e.g. as daughter, mother, wife, or partner.

In a group we will 'perform' a role in the way we have learned for a given situation, or in a way that is familiar to us, and according to our own given need or 'agenda'.

Activity

What role do you play within your class group?
Are you active as a leader or are you a team player? This could determine what role you are comfortable with as a member of a group.

Barriers to communication

Communication with other people is not always straightforward. There are factors which can be called *barriers to communication*, because they get in the way of our effective communication with others. The barriers may be to do with ourselves, the other person, or the interaction between us.

In communication terms:

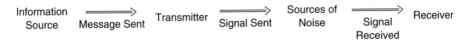

Figure 8.3   *The transmission of a message (Shannon and Weaver, 1949)*

In this model, the communication is not just one way (from sender to receiver) but forwarded on. In the course of transmission 'the message' may become confused or distorted.

Activity

Think of some examples of barriers to interpersonal communication.
   What gets in the way of your being able to communicate with another person?

There are a range of factors that you may have thought of such as:

- Not always immediately liking those people with whom we have to work.
- Having prejudices.
- Difficulty in understanding others.
- Someone may have a speech impediment.
- Someone has a hearing problem.

In addition there may be some problem with the environment in which the communication takes place:

- It is noisy.
- There is no privacy.
- There are distractions.

In some of these examples specialist skills may be required. You might be required as a care worker to gain some additional training and learn other forms of communication, such as MAKATON or British Sign Language. You may need extra training to understand better the need of the service user, e.g. dementia care, knowledge of autism, deaf awareness.
   In all of these situations you may need to be aware that your service user's experience is different from that of your own, especially if you have not come across the situation before. The person may have a range of different needs. The person may have English as a second language or may not speak English at all. In each of these cases you may need to use your own initiative to get the

help or training that you need. You should not be afraid to discuss your needs with someone at work, such as your supervisor, who will be pleased that you have identified this training need yourself.

Managing conflict situations

As you develop the work-related part of your Foundation Degree, you will increasingly come into contact with service users. It is likely that one of your main motivations for undertaking this particular course of study will be to help people or to work with a particular service user group. Working with others is not always 'plain sailing'. There may be times when the job is frustrating and when tensions creep into the work. Care work is in the top 10 of most stressful jobs, along with the police, the armed services, nursing and teaching. When people are stressed, they sometimes say and do things they wish they had not. Equally for the service users, their vulnerability means that they are also in stressful situations. The two factors combined can lead to potential conflict situations.

Being aware of the degree of stress you are under as either a student or a worker is important in monitoring your own stress levels. We all need a certain degree of stress in order to motivate ourselves in everyday situations. If we have too much stress we fall into 'eustress' or 'distress' – a level of stress, which, for us, is unhelpful. Everyone is different and not everyone experiences stress in the same way. When we are feeling like this and we are at work, we may be liable to 'fall out with' either the people we are working with, or maybe more likely the service users momentarily in an unhelpful way.

It is important therefore to be aware of the factors that can avert conflict and also how to manage conflict situations if they arise.

One way of looking at our behaviour is to consider our own individual conflict style. How do we approach situations? Are we aggressive, non-assertive or assertive? What do these words mean in relation to our behaviour?

How would you recognise a person who was being aggressive? They may be:

- Looking angry.
- Shouting.
- Tense.
- Flushed in the face.
- Glaring at somebody.
- Clenching their fist.
- Sarcastic.
- Unkind towards somebody.

It is most likely that when someone is behaving aggressively they want to be in control of a situation and feel they have to 'win' at all costs, whether it is the argument or another outcome. If this happens it will leave the other person in a 'lose' situation. In other words a positive outcome for the aggressor, but a negative outcome for the 'loser'. This is not the best outcome for either party.

What about someone who was non-assertive? They may:

- Be very tentative as they approach new situations.
- Speak quietly and apologetically.
- Find it difficult to stand up for themselves.
- Be unable to speak from their own point of view.

If a person behaves like this in a given situation, they will leave it feeling dissatisfied, confused and that no one has listened to them. They will certainly be unlikely to have gained what they wanted. A good example of the above would be getting served in a busy shop, complaining about a meal, being asked to change shift when it is not convenient. Many people, particularly women, find it hard to stand up for themselves and say 'no' when they think they might hurt people's feelings.

Assertiveness is the third 'conflict management' style. To assume this style is to be calm and confident in your approach, to be prepared to state your point of view, but prepared to negotiate. If you adopted this approach because you were not happy about your meal, you would be polite, ask for the waiter to give you a moment and then clearly state what you felt was wrong with your meal without apologising for it. It would go something like this:

> Excuse me. Could I have a word with you for a moment, please? *[Voice level]*
> This soup is cold.

The response should be:

> I'm very sorry; I'll replace it for you.

If you said 'I'm afraid the soup is cold' [*Apologetically*], it sounds as if you do not feel that you have the right to complain when your food is not the correct temperature.

Equally if you said aggressively 'This soup is cold. Can't you get the temperature right?' [*Sarcastically*], it would not help the waiter to continue to give you good service, because it would make him nervous and annoyed.

To summarise:
The best way to communicate in order to gain a satisfactory outcome for both parties and to avoid escalating a conflict is:

(Continued)

(Continued)

- To remain calm.
- State your point of view.
- Listen to the other person's point of view.
- Maintain eye contact.
- Have an open body posture.
- Be prepared to negotiate.

Use assertive behaviour to create a 'win–win' situation for both parties.

Here is an example in a care situation:

Elsie is an older service user in a residential home and has dementia. She becomes confused when dressing in the morning and requires assistance. The care worker is in a hurry because she has other residents to assist, and becomes impatient. The resident reacts by snatching away her skirt. The tension builds.

What should the care worker have done differently?

Be aware of the special requirements of Elsie as a woman with particular needs. That is:

- Allow her more time.
- Be patient.
- Promote her independence.
- Communicate with her supportively.
- Treat her with respect.

Elsie, like any older person, will be sensitive to the way her care is delivered and to the person who delivers it.

SUMMARY

Working with individuals and groups with effective communication skills is essential when working in health and social care. You need to be able to overcome the barriers of communication with the people you will be working with to provide an effective service to people. Interpersonal communication skills are the essential tool that you must have when working with people who may require your help and support. By reflecting on your use of communication skills you can continue with your personal and professional development by learning how to use effectively the core skills of empathy, listening and attending using SOLER and adopting a person-centred way of working. These essential skills will not only benefit the people you will be providing services to, but also benefit your other personal and professional relationships.

Further reading

Hargie, O. and Dickson, D. (2004) *Social Skills in Interpersonal Communication: research and practice,* 4th edn. London: Routledge. This is a good book because it provides a detailed overview of interpersonal communication covering many of the essential areas. You will be able to use it to develop further your interpersonal communication skills.

Johnson, D. and Johnson, F. (1998) *Joining Together: Group Theory and Group Skills.* London: Prentice Hall. If you are interested in working with groups of people this is a key text for understanding communication in groups.

9 PLANNING AND MANAGING CARE

Graham Brotherton

SUMMARY CHAPTER CONTENTS

- Assessment issues

  (a) Defining need
  (b) Financial assessment
  (c) Eligibility criteria
  (d) Approaches to assessment

- Care management issues

  (a) Defining care or case management
  (b) Assessment and empowerment
  (c) Service brokerage
  (d) Risk and assessment

Learning objectives

By the end of this chapter, you should be able to:

■ Outline different ways of thinking about the concept of need.

■ Describe and evaluate approaches to assessment.

■ Evaluate the usefulness of different approaches to care or case management.

Introduction – thinking about needs

Central to the justification for health and social care services, and indeed of welfare services more generally, is the claim that they are meeting the 'needs' of individuals or groups. However, the concept of need is not a straightforward one; for example, can someone ever 'need' cosmetic surgery, or how far should the state go in meeting the needs of those who have 'chosen' not to work? Need is therefore closely related to both values and ideology. This is significant because the way in which need is conceptualised has significant implications for the way in which services will be provided.

There have been several attempts to conceptualise 'need' in ways that are relevant to health and social care. One of the earliest and still among the best known is the model developed by Bradshaw. He suggested that 'needs' can be defined in four ways:

- Normative – need as defined by 'professionals'.
- Felt – individual's wants, wishes or desires.
- Expressed – verbal 'requests' or the way in which people use services.
- Comparative – relating the needs of one group to those in similar circumstances or situations.

Activity

This might seem a little abstract, but try to think of a person or care situation you are familiar with. How might looking at need from these four different 'angles' influence the way the person or situation is viewed?

One of the key consequences of thinking about need in this way is that we can begin to think about whose 'need' it is. Should we prioritise professional perceptions over those of service users or should we always give precedence to user perspectives – how can we reconcile the different points of view?

A different approach to conceptualising need was developed by Doyal and Gough (1991) who argue that there are some basic 'human needs' which are universal and apply to everyone regardless of their individual circumstances. They argue that in complex societies where rights, responsibilities and duties are allocated as a condition of social participation, then individuals are entitled to have their needs met to a level which enables them to participate and discharge their social responsibilities and duties. Doyal and Gough see entitlements which stem from this as being linked to both health and autonomy, central concerns of health and social care practice. They go on to develop a case which highlights the way in which relativist critiques of universal rights are usually internally inconsistent and that other objections to universal needs based on cultural or diversity arguments often overlook similarities in the ways in which key needs, e.g. the need to be healthy, are conceptualised. Doyal and Gough's work is given a new resonance if we compare some of their arguments with the New Labour model of rights and responsibilities in welfare provision. In the New Labour model rights are to some extent at least conditional on the discharge of responsibilities (e.g. through the 'New Deal' approach to work and benefit where entitlement to benefit is linked to the requirement to be actively seeking work). For Doyal and Gough, though, the link is one of entitlement rather than conditionality.

Another writer who has attempted to take a universalist approach is Nussbaum. Using an argument that is similar to the one developed by Doyal and Gough she suggests that there are 10 'Central Functional Human Capabilities' which are for our purposes the same as human needs. These are (Nussbaum, 2000: 78–80):

- Life as in a 'normal' lifespan.
- Bodily health – to be healthy and have access to the necessities which support health, namely food, shelter, etc.
- Bodily integrity – including freedom of movement, being secure against all forms of violence and assault, the ability to express sexuality.
- Senses, imagination and thought – encompassing literacy, freedom of expression (creatively, politically and spiritually).
- Emotions – the ability to love and care and to have this reciprocated.
- Practical reason – the ability to reflect upon and be involved in the planning of one's own life.
- Affiliation – the ability to live with and associate with others (including support for the social and political institutions which support this).
- Other species – living with and showing concern for other species.
- Play – being able to laugh and enjoy recreation.
- Control over one's political (both micro and macro) and material environments.

Activity

To what extent do services you are familiar with either as a worker or service user support Nussbaum's 'Central Functional Human Capabilities'?

Do you agree that all of the 'capabilities' are important? (You might want to think about other statements of rights like the UN Conventions on Human Rights and Children's Rights.)

How well do your assessment and care management processes support all of the capabilities?

There are of course problems with any model which attempts to develop an approach which claims to be transferable across time and cultures, though both Doyal and Gough and Nussbaum do emphasise that the processes of identifying needs and capabilities are dynamic and likely to be reflected in different ways in different contexts. Nonetheless, as practitioners involved in decisions about 'who gets what' it is vital to be able to locate these decisions in the broader context of views about rights and entitlements.

Assessment and care management in the UK

As outlined in Chapter 6, the history of assessment and care management in the UK can be traced back to the 'casework' approach as developed by the Charity Organisation Society in the second half of the nineteenth century. This model has shaped the subsequent development of practice with its emphases on the 'facts' of a situation and on eligibility and whether the recipient is perceived as 'deserving'.

This remains an issue of importance, in that when we are considering access to health and social care services in the UK, we need to acknowledge that there are two ways in which we assess eligibility: through financial assessment and through eligibility criteria.

Financial assessment

While access to health care services is free at the time that we use them (though we all contribute to the cost of health care through National Insurance and thorough general taxation), access to social care services is 'means tested'. At the point at which someone is assessed in terms of their need for services, they also go for a financial assessment which determines their ability to contribute to the cost of their own care. As a result of changes introduced as part of the 'Fairer Access to Care Services' initiative (explained in more detail in the later section on eligibility) costs are now broadly similar across all local authorities, though the charging system is quite complicated. Most local authorities include details of their charging policy in the health and social care information sections of their web sites.

Activity

Look at the information available on some local authority web sites.

Do you think the system would be clear to a person newly requiring care or their carer?

Do the charging policies seem 'fair' to you?

Eligibility

One of the most complex issues in looking at assessment and case or care management is the issue of eligibility. Implicit in any assessment process is a decision or decisions about entitlement to services. In this sense anyone acting as an 'assessor' is acting as a 'gatekeeper', making decisions about who will or will not gain access to services and under what conditions. There are a number of factors which are of significance in considering eligibility:

- **Resources:** In most cases the total number of people who could benefit from a service will be greater than the capacity of the service. Decisions therefore need to be made about who will gain most benefit (however this is conceptualised) from the service.
- **Geography:** In most case services are not evenly distributed, especially more specialised services; there are therefore issues about access based upon where you live. Even where services exist there may be differences between gatekeepers and their employing authorities in terms of their willingness to pay for access to services.
- **Attitudes:** This operates on at least two levels. Firstly in respect of general social attitudes, some groups may be seen as more 'deserving' than others, leading to some groups experiencing difficulty in accessing resources, e.g. those who have misused drugs or alcohol. On a second level those carrying out the assessment will themselves approach the assessment process with particular preconceptions that can influence that process. An example here (Katbamna et al., 2002) would be that there is evidence that assumptions about the existence of extended families which provide support can lead to services not being offered to some South Asian service users or carers.
- **Criteria:** Most assessment processes work to pre-set criteria which attempt to provide a structure for dealing with the issues highlighted above. However, the sheer complexity inherent with dealing with the range of factors that can influence the assessment process will make administration of any assessment a highly skilled task.

Activity

Look at some Social Services Department web sites. In most you will find explanations of the assessment criteria used within the authority.

What sort of criteria are used?

How effective do you think they are likely to be in ensuring that services go to those who need them most?

Since the introduction of the 'Fair Access to Care Services' (Department of Health, 2003a) approach, which was a response to a suggested 'postcode lottery' in terms of both availability and cost, criteria have become much more similar with all local authorities required to use four levels of need: critical, substantial, moderate and low. The criteria from the original document are reproduced in the box below. In most cases resources are concentrated on providing services for people who fall into the first two categories, with some allocation for people who fall into the third. While looking at the criteria you might want to think about how easy it might be to use the criteria in order to place people in each of the levels and about whether people in the lower two categories 'should' gain access to services given that using the criteria they may still have very real support needs.

Level 1	Critical	• life is, or will be, threatened; • significant health problems have developed or will develop; • there is, or will be, little or no choice and control over vital aspects of the immediate environment; • serious abuse or neglect has occurred or will occur; • there is, or will be, an inability to carry out vital personal care or domestic routines; • vital involvement in work, education or learning cannot or will not be sustained; • vital social support systems and relationships cannot or will not be sustained; • vital family and other social roles and responsibilities cannot or will not be undertaken.
Level 2	Substantial	• there is, or will be, only partial choice and control over the immediate environment; and/or • abuse or neglect has occurred or will occur; and/or • there is, or will be, an inability to carry out the majority of personal care or domestic routines; and/or • involvement in many aspects of work, education or learning cannot or will not be sustained; and/or • the majority of social support systems and relationships cannot or will not be sustained; and/or • the majority of family and other social roles and responsibilities cannot or will not be undertaken.
Level 3	Moderate	• there is, or will be, an inability to carry out several personal care or domestic routines; and/or • involvement in several aspects of work, education or learning cannot or will not be sustained; and/or • several social support systems and relationships cannot or will not be sustained; and/or

(Continued)

(Continued)	
Level 4 Low	• several family and other social roles and responsibilities cannot or will not be undertaken. • there is, or will be, an inability to carry out one or two personal care or domestic routines; and/or • involvement in one or two aspects of work, education or learning cannot or will not be sustained; and/or • one or two social support systems and relationships cannot or will not be sustained; and/or • one or two family and other social roles and responsibilities cannot or will not be undertaken.

There have been moves towards the development of multi-agency approaches to assessment with the development of single assessment approaches to be shared by a range of professionals. This can be seen in fullest form in the development of the Common Assessment Framework (CAF) as part of Every Child Matters and the Children Act 2004. This is a single form which can be filled in by any one of a range of workers involved with a child and utilises a common format for each; details can be found at www.ecm.gov.uk/caf. The CAF has been used on a trial basis in a number of areas and will be a national requirement by April 2008.

The single assessment process

The way in which adults who need health and social care services are assessed is currently undergoing revision with the introduction of the single assessment process. This approach, which was introduced as part of the National Service Framework for Older People, is an integrated approach to multiple assessments where the various professionals might carry out an assessment as part of an overall assessment process, e.g. social workers, occupational therapists, etc.

The process has four stages:

- Initial contact assessment
- Overview assessment
- In-depth/specialist assessment
- Comprehensive assessment.

The initial and overview assessment are completed by the service that someone initially comes into contact with. The various in-depth/specialist assessments will be specific to each organisation which might become involved. As assessments for older people comprise the bulk of health and social care assessments, most assessments will be carried out using the single assessment process. It must, though, be pointed out that at this point there is no nationally agreed format for carrying out the single assessment process nor is there any form of integrated IT system to support the process (though this is planned). As a result there may be considerable variations in the way in which the single assessment process operates in different areas, though these are likely to diminish over time as the central IT systems develop.

However, for other people who require support there will still be a range of approaches. For example, the Care Programme Approach will still be used for mental health assessments and the Person-Centred Planning Approach for people with learning disabilities.

Activity

Look at the assessment documents for your own agency and try to find details for other agencies (some local authorities have quite a lot of detail on their web sites, for example).

Try to identify:

o The general approach that is being used.
o Whose 'interests' are being prioritised.

Approaches to assessment

In most cases assessment is seeking to achieve a number of different things, some of which may be awkward to reconcile with each other. In this section a couple of key dimensions of assessment will be explored. Firstly, types of assessment will be considered. There are broadly speaking two general approaches to assessment, functional and holistic, though these are better considered as opposite poles of a continuum rather than completely separate approaches. Functional assessment is concerned with what a person can or cannot 'do' as an individual and often attempts to categorise this in particular ways, e.g. self-care. Holistic assessment attempts to locate people in their particular context, the physical and social environment that they are in, etc., and is concerned with the relationship between the person and their environments.

Whilst in practice most assessments comprise elements of both, it is important to consider the balance between the two. In the final chapter you will look at the medical and social models of disability and while not wishing to oversimplify the debate it can be seen that the holistic assessment is more easily compatible with the social model and vice versa. There is, though, a second element to this, in that there is also the issue of 'ownership' of the assessment process. Assessment is partly about identifying the 'needs' of service users and their carers, partly about 'eligibility' as discussed earlier, both in terms of general access to services and also 'suitability' for specific services. In other words, assessment is about meeting the needs of a variety of 'stakeholders'.

The key 'stakeholders' in the assessment process are the service user (or in the case of initial assessment, the potential service user), the carer, the Social Services Department or other funding body, and the service provider or providers.

Activity

Think about the assessment process from the functional and holistic perspectives outlined above:

o What would be your key concerns?
o What might you hope to 'obtain' from the assessment process?
o Whose interests do you think are likely to be prioritised?

While every situation is unique, the sorts of things you might have thought about might include the service user wanting to obtain a flexible and responsive range of services, whereas the Social Services Department needs to consider the funding of this; the carer wanting a slightly different range of services from the service user and having his or her own distinctive needs (e.g. for some form of respite from the caring role); and the service provider wanting to be able to provide services in ways which 'fit' with its own capacity and priorities.

In this sense we need to recognise that assessment is a contested process and that some of the disparate interests identified above may not always be easily reconciled. In thinking about whose interests are prioritised, again we need to recognise that there is a complicated process of negotiation which links to earlier discussions about the role of professional power (see Chapters 4 and 5).

Carer's assessment

One way in which some of the issues discussed above have been recognised is through the introduction of a notionally separate assessment process for carers. Whilst there has been a process in place since the early 1990s there have been two pieces of legislation: the Carers and Disabled Children Act 2000 and the Carers (Equal Opportunities) Act 2004, which strengthen the requirement to identify carers' needs separately and to provide greater support specifically focused on carers. The Carers UK web site provides a very useful overview.

There has also been some recognition of the very specific issues which face young carers and a number of initiatives have been developed to support the estimated 150,000 children and young people who are primary carers (further information can be found on individual local authority web sites in terms of how these services are arranged locally).

There is, though, still some evidence that carers are not always assessed in an appropriate way. Scourfield (2005), in a very clear summary drawing on earlier work by Twigg and Atkin (1994), provides a clear overview of possible explanations for this. He suggests that carers are viewed by professionals in one of four ways:

- 'Co-workers'. In this view carers are active participants in the care of the person they are providing care for and are viewed as such by local authorities. Their role is largely perceived as benign, but this role is rarely recognised in its own right; they are seen only in the context of the relationship with the 'cared-for' person. In this sense it can obscure the often intricate relationship which exists and especially the potential for 'abuse' in this context. Scourfield suggests this is the default perception of carers from many professionals.
- 'Co-clients'. In this view the carers are seen as a 'client' in their own right and separate needs are more likely to be addressed, leading to a more open discussion of possible tensions between the 'carer' and 'cared for', though it may also create the problem of a failure to acknowledge fully the specific needs of the person receiving care.
- The 'carers as a resource' model could be said to reflect the dominant models of health and social care. In this model carers are perceived only in relation to the role that they perform and no differentiation is made between different types of informal carers (family, friends, etc.) and their specific relationship to the person receiving care. As a result of this informal carers are unlikely to be offered carers' assessment.
- The final category, the 'superseded carer', refers to situations where the carer's role has been replaced by the provision of formal services. In this situation there has been a clear separation of both roles and interests and potential conflicts are fully recognised. In many circumstances the term carer ceases to be used and is replaced by the use of 'family' or 'relative'.

Scourfield goes on to argue the case for greater clarity in terms of the way that carers are perceived as a basis for a more open approach to negotiating questions of need. This example provides a useful insight into the issues around recognising the needs of particular stakeholders and the possible tensions which can occur within the assessment process.

Care management

If someone finds their way through the assessment process and becomes entitled to receipt of services they then enter the care or case management process. This refers to the process of identifying and monitoring the provision of services within a 'mixed economy of care'. Current approaches date back to the idea of case management which emerged in the 1980s. The idea of 'case management' was to provide an individualised system in which care was based upon individual need as identified by a lead professional or professionals. This term is undergoing something of a revival in the health context, especially in the context of community services.

What is case/care management?

The terms case and care management are not always easy to define as the following extract from 'Case management competences framework for the care of people with long term conditions' (Department of Health, 2005) illustrates:

> Case management in both the NHS and social care does not have a generally accepted common definition or shared language between the many professionals involved and this can cause confusion when trying to organise a service or when developing the workforce. At the heart of the case management competences framework is the need to be proactive and co-ordinated in identifying the most complex and vulnerable people with a long term condition and then co-ordinating and managing their care in partnership with the individual and their carers. There are several models operating successfully and many health and social care professionals are involved.

Skills for Health (2005) have produced a diagram (see Figure 9.1) which attempts to look at how 'case management' as a model applies in health and social care contexts.

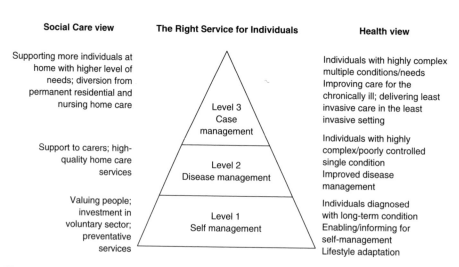

Figure 9.1

A third 'angle' on case/care management can be found in the 'Guidance on Delivering Services and Multi Agency Working (2005)' on the DfES 'Every Child Matters' web site. This suggests a three stage Process;

1   Preparation – gathering information about the 'case', identifying concerns, talking to key individuals, carrying out or arranging for the carrying out of an assessment (in this case the CAF).
2   Discussion of the 'results' of the assessment process leading where appropriate to single- or multi-agency support – at this stage a 'lead professional' is involved.
3   Service delivery – implementation of agreed actions on a 'plan, do and review' basis monitored by a lead professional.

Activity

Think about how the models above apply to people you work with or are familiar with.
  o Do you see 'case management' in action?
  o What are its strengths and weaknesses as an approach?

Case management or care management?

Perhaps the most useful way of making the distinction between the two is to see 'case management' as a general term for the planning and co-ordinating of care and to use 'care management' to refer specifically to the process used for assessing and managing care as set out in the National Health Service and Community Care Act 1990. In this process the term care management incorporates the assessment of need, the financial assessment and the determination of eligibility implied in the Act and the subsequent Gloucestershire judgment (as outlined in Chapter 6). The other key component of the care management process is that where someone is identified as both having needs and being eligible for support, this leads to the development of a 'care package' which is a co-ordinated range of services (or in some cases a single service) designed to meet those needs. A couple of points of clarification are required here. Firstly, this does not mean that all identified needs have to be met; as mentioned previously, the local authority is also charged with balancing its community care budget. Secondly, a key component of this model is the existence of a range of care agencies able to provide services in the context of a 'mixed economy'.

Assessment and empowerment

It is in this process of assessment and care/case management that some of the issues around power and empowerment can be seen most explicitly. As explained at the start of this chapter, assessment serves a number of potentially conflicting purposes, in terms for example of prioritising access to services through the use of eligibility criteria mediating different conceptions of need between competing stakeholders. This potentially sits uncomfortably with the expressed aim of policy which has been to create greater flexibility and choice for users of care services. This is illustrated by the statement of aims from the Green Paper, 'Independence, Well-being and Choice' (Department of Health, 2005).

Over the next 10 to 15 years, we want to work with people who use social care to help them transform their lives by:

* ensuring they have more control;
* giving them more choices and helping them decide how their needs can best be met;
* giving them the chance to do the things that other people take for granted;
* giving the best quality of support and protection to those with the highest levels of need.

The proposals in the Green Paper include a number which are of note in terms of the way in which assessment and care management might develop. The first is the area of self-assessment, which is the idea that people may be able to assess themselves, possibly through some form of online self-assessment questionnaire for access to simple services. How this might work in practice and the limits to what a 'simple service' might be are not as yet clear.

The second strand looks likely to be an extension of the direct payments approach. While direct payments have been around since the Community Care (Direct Payments) Act 1996, the number of people utilising them has been small (the Green Paper suggests that in 2003 about 12,500 of the 1.7 million people who use care services were using direct payments). Since April 2003 a change in regulations means that local authorities have to inform people who use care services that they are entitled to direct payments, though it is not yet clear whether this has led to a significant increase in the number of applicants.

The principle of direct payments is that following assessment the person who needs support is given a sum of money to purchase the support that they need. There are some limitations on how the money can be spent (e.g. purchasing care from a close relative is prohibited) and a requirement to keep records of spending, but the principle is that it creates greater flexibility in terms of how the person can choose to organise their own support and that power is moved form service providers to the person using the services.

Some of the reasons which have been suggested for the slow uptake of direct payments have been: difficulty in finding information about who can provide services, the complications associated with effectively becoming an employer (of those that provide support) and the fact that many vulnerable people might find it problematic to take on this role. In response to this there has been an increased recognition of the role that service brokerage might play in developing the direct payments approach (see next section). The Green Paper proposes that direct payments could in principle by extended through the use of agents. This means that where a person is felt not to be able to consent to or be able to manage a direct payment (e.g. as a result of dementia) then someone could be nominated by the local authority to manage a payment on their behalf – possibly a spouse or other family member. This will operate in the context of the new mental capacity legislation due to come into force in 2007.

Service (or support) brokerage

This model, which originated in Canada as service brokerage, has been receiving increasing support in recent years. Its basic premise is that an intermediary is used to help a person locate and access services which are appropriate to them. In the UK the Commission for Social Care Inspection in its discussion document on brokerage and its possible applicability uses the term support brokerage. In practice the two terms are largely synonymous. In their paper 'Support Brokerage: A Discussion Paper', CSCI (2006) suggests that the role of a support broker would be to work under the direction of the person requiring support and possibly carers to:

- access an assessment of their care needs;
- select or put together a care plan which fits their needs;
- obtain or negotiate and manage funding to pay for the care service;
- implement the plans;
- monitor and evaluate the service;
- build personal networks;
- mediate and resolve problems; and
- provide help and advice as long as the person uses care services.

There are a number of possible models in terms of how brokerage could be put into practice and a number of significant issues to be resolved, e.g. should brokers work inside or outside the existing system? How would brokerage be paid for?

Activity

For a fuller discussion of the issues raised in this section see the CSCI web site, http://www.csci.org.uk.

How might the introduction of a service brokerage approach affect you and the people you work with?

The Green Paper on the future of services for children who are 'looked after', namely 'Care Matters: Transforming the Lives of Children and Young People in Care' (DfES, 2006), advocates a variant of this with children being given an individual budget which will be administered through a new range of independent social work practices analogous to GP practices, though at the time of writing it is unclear as to whether this proposal will ultimately become reality.

The role of risk and accountability in the assessment process

One of the other key debates in health and social care which is clearly illustrated by the assessment and care management process is the role of risk. At the heart of any discussion is the balance between providing appropriate 'protection' for vulnerable people and the need to support people's autonomy and provide genuine opportunities to support independence, individuality and growth. Once again this creates tensions within the process with the need for the assessor to demonstrate 'safe' decisions and thereby satisfy the demands of accountability being in possible conflict with the aspirations of the service user for greater flexibility. It has to be borne in mind that developmental activity with some groups of people who use care services is both essential to good practice and inherently 'risky'. To give a couple of examples, supporting people's autonomy by enabling people either to use public transport independently, or to pursue personal relationships, would both be considered good practice, but raise considerable issues about identifying and managing risk which can lead to excessively cautious approaches being taken. As highlighted previously in the discussion of the fair access to care criteria, risk is also a central component of the assessment and care management process in that it is one of the criteria which influence eligibility for services.

A further manifestation of these issues can be seen in the area of abuse, the identification of which is central to any assessment process. While some categories of abuse, e.g. the sexual abuse of young children or physical abuse in formal care settings, are clear cut, many others are more complex. For example, when does poor parenting become child neglect or the increasing stress or tension linked to caring for a long-term partner who has dementia become abusive? The current frameworks around protecting vulnerable people are for adults those introduced by *No Secrets* (Department of Health, 2000) and *Working together to safeguard children* (DfES, 2006). Every agency should have policies which deal with protection and it is important to be aware of the policy which applies in any agency in which you are working.

This all takes place in the context of a system in which there is an increased emphasis on 'accountability' in the sense of a requirement to be able to justify actions and decisions in resource, practice and financial terms. This has arisen as a direct response to both the demand for more efficient services which has been at the heart of most of the reforms of health and social care and the perceived failure of services to deliver appropriate support and protection in a number of high-profile cases. The implications of accountability are discussed more fully in the final chapter.

New Labour reforms

In the White Paper *Our health, our care, our say* (Department of Health, 2006) the government set out its current thinking in a number of areas which are likely to have far-reaching implications for the future of health and social care services; the broader implications are considered in the next chapter. In this context the paper proposes a shift to a more person-centred model of services based on greater individual choice; this is illustrated by the quote below:

> Services should be personcentred, seamless and proactive. They should support independence, not dependence and allow everyone to enjoy a good quality of life, including the ability to contribute fully to our communities. They should treat people with respect and dignity and support them in overcoming barriers to inclusion. They should be tailored to the religious, cultural and ethnic needs of individuals. They should focus on positive outcomes and well-being, and work proactively to include the most disadvantaged groups. We want to ensure that everyone, particularly people in the most excluded groups in our society, benefits from improvements in services.

There are, though, some crucial questions here about how this will operate in the context of a move to, on the one hand, greater use of the mixed economy and the private sector and, on the other, the move to multi-agency working and joined-up services.

SUMMARY

Perhaps the most significant issue to be raised in this chapter is that of the complexity of the assessment process and the way that differing 'stakeholders' in the process are likely to have different expectations and aspirations which are influenced by their role within the process. Key factors and issues which affect this are:

- Key concepts which are often used as if they have accepted shared meanings but in fact are often contested, such as the concept of need.

- In some areas such as the care management process there is again some uncertainty as to the precise meaning of key policy terms and hence some ambiguity about how to put process into practice.

- Service users, carers and the various workers involved may have very different priorities which are heavily influenced by their personal or professional circumstances.

Review questions ?

- How can we make sure that the assessment process recognises and takes account of the interests of the various 'stakeholders' involved even where this may create tension or uncertainty?
- What are the implications of key policy changes such as the move to direct payments and brokerage likely to be for health and social care practitioners?
- How will this be influenced by the mixed economy approach and the move to multi-agency working?

Further reading

MacDonald, A. (2006) *Understanding Community Care: A Guide for Social Workers*. London: Palgrave Macmillan. A clear and accessible guide to the issues covered in this chapter from a social work perspective.

Doyal, L. and Gough, I. (1991) *A Theory of Human Need*. London: Palgrave Macmillan. A challenging book, but it provides a compelling case for a universalist approach to services and a point of comparison with the emphasis on 'needs-led' or 'targeted' approaches set out in this chapter.

10 THE FUTURE OF HEALTH AND SOCIAL CARE SERVICES

Graham Brotherton

As we reach the end of this book it is important to take stock of the current picture with regard to health and social care in general, but also to look at workforce issues and the implications that this might have as you reach the end of your course. The current picture is complex with a process of rapid change meaning that the health and social care sector in 10 years' time is likely to be very different from the one of 10 years ago. In order to look at this, three major themes will be considered:

- The changing policy and practice context.
- The role of technology in shaping the future development of services.
- The changing health and social care workforce.

Inevitably a chapter on where things are going has to be a little speculative, though as highlighted in previous chapters there are a range of very clear 'clues' as to the future direction of services.

Activity

Using the three themes above, what seem to you to be the main 'issues'?
How has the way you work changed over the past few years in response to these issues?
How do you think it will change over the next few years?
What are the main implications for workers in health and social care services?

You might want to look again at your answers again at the end of the chapter and compare your thoughts with ours.

Policy and practice issues

Before returning in a bit more detail to the changing policy and practice context, it is worth looking a little more broadly at the way in which society itself has changed and the implications that this might have for the future of welfare services. The start point for this has to be that we live in an ageing society and that older people are the main users of health and social care services. Life expectancy in the UK has risen significantly in the last half century and the birth rate has fallen. As a result the balance of the population has significantly altered, though it is worth pointing out that these changes are not happening as quickly or dramatically in the UK as in many other European countries. This has very significant implications in that the welfare system has to a considerable extent worked on the assumption that the generation currently working will pay through taxes and National Insurance for the services required by the generation who have retired. As retirement has become longer and the number of people working as a proportion of the total population has fallen, this has led to a perceived crisis of funding. This is most obvious in terms of the current debate about the future of pensions, but it applies equally to health and care services.

In effect, in recent years the way in which this has been addressed is through the increased means testing of services which has led to a number of key policy consequences: firstly the increasing number of older people who are reliant on means-tested benefits to 'top-up' the state pension and secondly the number of older people who have to sell their home in order to pay for the costs of residential care.

In addition, as referred to in Chapter 6, there has been an increased debate on the future of the NHS and health care funding more generally, with the call from a number of sources for the introduction of a social insurance model.

Activity

Would the introduction of 'up front' charging and social insurance be a good way forward? What are the principal arguments for and against?

The Joseph Rowntree Foundation has done a lot of work looking at possible ways of funding social care for older people which summarises the arguments well (www.jrf.org.uk; look in the 'findings' section).

Social insurance, which is widely used in mainland Europe, is a system in which there is a more explicit link between contributions and access to services. For example, in France, which has often been used as a 'model' for good health services in recent years, both employer and employee pay a contribution to an independent insurance scheme run by a board on which both employers and trade unions have significant representation. As an example, people seeing a doctor pay up front and then claim back a proportion of the cost (around 75 per cent). There is also a facility for people to make extra contributions and claim a higher level of benefits/services and around 90 per cent of the population do this. The majority of European countries have systems based on variants of this model and supporters suggest that it has two very significant advantages. Firstly it can enable greater direct contributions from service users or potential service users perhaps creating a greater sense of ownership of services. Secondly it is sometimes argued that the use of 'up front' charges would encourage people to think more carefully about using services thus reducing inappropriate use of services (e.g. GP appointments).

The main complications or arguments against are around how you build in a 'safety net' for those who are unable to make contributions or whose contributions are insufficient to meet the costs of care, especially care in later life once someone has retired and is no longer making contributions. One solution used in Germany is to use the contributions of members of the wider family to meet the costs of the care of older people.

Globalisation, 'Third Way' politics and the repositioning of welfare

In the chapters which explored the social and legal context of health and social care services, the idea that health and social care services take place in a political and ideological context was introduced. As you reach the end of this book it is important to look at how this context is currently evolving. One of the central claims of this government has been that it represents a 'new' approach to politics – a 'Third Way' (the term has been used as a book title by both Tony Blair and Anthony Giddens, the sociologist whose ideas have heavily influenced the New Labour approach) – which is neither right nor left in the traditional sense. Central to Third Way politics is a belief that the world that we live in has changed fundamentally as a result of globalisation. While globalisation is a complex and multifaceted set of issues, it can be summarised as greater interconnectedness between nation-states in a variety of ways:

- Economic – the rapid movement of jobs and financial resources.
- Social – increased movement of people through both migration and tourism.
- Technologically – through the use of communication technology, computers, mobile phones, etc.

Globalisation also acknowledges that there is a changing balance between large global corporations and nation-states in that some of the largest corporations now have a turnover gross domestic product (the amount of money produced by a country) of greater than the most of the countries in the world.

Activity

How might each of these issues influence the development of health and social care services over the next few years?

Some examples might include:

- Economic – as welfare services are largely tax funded is it possible to maintain the 'flow' of resources as companies (and perhaps individuals) can move their financial resources rapidly around the globe?
- Social – this might include providing appropriate services in an increasingly multi-cultural society and issues about the recruitment and training of staff both from the diverse communities of the UK and from those who might have come from a variety of places to work in the British health and social care system. Some of the issues which arise from this are discussed more fully later in this chapter.
- Technology – using cameras to provide remote surveillance of vulnerable people; some nurseries already provide 'web-cams' so that parents can watch their children during the day. It has been suggested that this sort of technology could be used to support vulnerable older people. What do you think?

As a result of globalisation and other factors it is argued that people's lives in the west have become less predictable. The certainty that characterised the lives of most people, especially in the period after the Second World War when people's lives were 'mapped out' by social context, has largely disappeared. For most men in the post-war era this meant working in the same occupation for most of their lives; for women it meant being primarily perceived as a wife and mother. For most people it also meant living in the same geographical area for all of their lives. While for individuals this was clearly very constraining in terms of the organisation of welfare, it made planning of services easier in the sense that it was possible to make certain assumptions, especially about women's availability to provide informal care both for children and for older relatives. This was a central premise of the post-war Beveridge system.

The massive social changes of the past 40 years have had a profound influence on the assumptions made here. Changes in women's patterns of employment and changing family structures have combined with the decline of the large-scale manufacturing economy on which the Beveridge model was premised to create a world very different from the one the system was designed for. The idea of a 'job for life' for example now seems a very dated one with most people expecting to change not just jobs but also quite probably careers several times during their working lives.

However, these changes have not impacted upon everyone evenly. According to Giddens (2000), the 'risks' associated with these changes (e.g. the risk of long-term unemployment) have fallen disproportionately on particular groups of people who often feel that they have little ability to resist change. An example might be people living in a town dependent on a single large employer who find that their jobs have been moved to another part of the world leaving them with very limited employment prospects. This process can lead to people feeling passive and perceiving themselves to be unable to deal with the circumstances they find themselves in. This is taking place in the context of significant demographic changes as described in the last section. It means that there is in practice an increased demand for people of working age to be working (especially when, as in the UK in recent years, this is combined with economic growth which itself leads to a greater demand for workers). A central purpose of the welfare system needs therefore to contribute to maximising the available supply of workers.

The welfare 'system' therefore needs to be able to create the circumstances in which people will be able to take some measure of control of their own lives through a combination of training and benefits designed either to 'encourage' or 'coerce' people into looking for work depending upon your viewpoint. This includes an emphasis on encouraging people who have been historically excluded from work, such as many people with disabilities.

Moving to a social model for health and social care?

Another significant trend which links to the issues discussed in the previous section has been a move towards thinking about both disability and illness in different ways. As outlined in Chapter 4, there are tensions in the way in which both disease and disability are conceptualised by differing groups. A useful way of exploring this is through the social and medical models.

The medical model focuses on abnormalities or limitations within the person, which require expert diagnosis and either 'cure' or management by those with expert knowledge, in this context usually doctors. The focus is the 'disease' or 'condition' and on the specialist knowledge and services required to manage this. This often requires the use of specialised services which may be segregated and require the 'approval' of a professional gatekeeper in order to gain access. The responsibility for adjustment lies with the individual who is expected to adapt to 'fit in' with existing social structures.

The social model focuses on the way in which social situations or structures contribute to excluding those with either a disability or a limiting illness. In this model disability is a combination of individual impairment and social attitudes. An obvious example of this process is the way in which physical environments have often been designed to meet the needs of younger, physically fit people and can inhibit many others, be they older people, people with disabilities or parents attempting to push young children in buggies. Supporters of the social model highlight the fact that professional power has been a significant factor in defining the way in which disability is thought about or 'constructed', and argue that progress can only be made through the changing of attitudes and the creation of inclusive services open to all, for example, through a genuinely 'inclusive' education system.

A useful insight into this process is provided by the ideas of Michel Foucault who argued (though it is important to acknowledge that this is oversimplifying the argument somewhat, see for example Turner, 1995) that as religion had declined as a way of providing a moral framework for living during the Enlightenment, this role was picked up by science and the emerging medical profession. An example of this can be found in Chapter 6 and the notion of classification which underpinned both the workhouse system and the subsequent emergence of the institutions. One of the major classifications was that of 'moral defective', a catch-all category which included women who became pregnant outside marriage and those who committed crimes such as theft. Many writers, especially from the disability movements, have highlighted the way in which the legacy of this approach continues both attitudes and services; again the debate around 'inclusive' versus 'specialist' education can be seen as an illustration of this.

Surveillance versus empowerment

A further dimension of this debate concerns one of the central tensions of health and social care practice. Care services are expected both to support those 'in need' and to regulate those who are perceived to have behaved in ways which are seen as 'wrong' or unacceptable. This balance plays out in different ways in different parts of the health and social care sector, so for example in child protection the emphasis is very much on the latter, in some (but by no means all) adult social care services the emphasis is on the former and in other areas, e.g. mental health services, both aspects are explicitly present. This places front line workers in often difficult positions in that they can be simultaneously expected to act in both supportive and coercive ways. This can be seen as a continuation of the moral surveillance described by Foucault whereby practitioners can be seen as policing acceptability in terms of particular aspects of behaviour, e.g. attitudes to seeking work or parenting practice.

There is, though, a further dimension to the surveillance debate: some commentators have argued that one of the defining features of health and social care practice in general but perhaps of social care practice in particular has been 'deprofessionalisation', which can be defined as a reduction of the amount of discretion given to practitioners to make professional judgements and the introduction of greater levels of scrutiny of day-to-day practice. This has its roots both in the various inquiries which have criticised the quality of social care practice, of which the most recent and perhaps most significant is the Laming Report into the death of Victoria Climbie (Department of Health, 2003b) and in the reforms of the 1980s onwards with the introduction of managerialist approaches which emphasise the achievement of externally defined targets.

For younger or newer practitioners it is perhaps worth pointing out that the idea of independent inspectorates (described in more detail in Chapter 6) is a relatively new one and not a model which is widely used internationally. In many other countries ideas about professional discretion and peer review of practice remain the dominant models, though it has to be acknowledged that the debate about how best to ensure good practice and professional accountability is an ongoing one in most welfare systems.

Activity

How far should practitioners be involved in the process of 'surveillance'? Are there occasions when this is important? What do you perceive as the dangers and how can workers and organisations set boundaries on their role?

In contrast to this, how far should we go in monitoring the actions of practitioners: do you think inspection promotes or hinders good practice?

One of the major problems which can be associated with the rise of inspection and accountability is the tendency to develop defensive models of practice. This means a model of working which involves 'playing safe' in terms of the way we work with people and an emphasis on formal record keeping as a basis for the justification of a particular approach or intervention. While there are clearly some important benefits to this model and we would all wish for example for our GP to practise safely when prescribing medication, there may be drawbacks in some situations. Much health and social care work has an explicitly developmental function which involves the managed taking of risks. In the context of defensive practice it may be that we find ourselves taking an overly cautious approach because of concerns about accountability, which may not be in the service users' best interests. This is obviously a difficult area but one to which practitioners need to give considerable thought.

As outlined in the previous chapter, one of the key apparent drivers of health and social care policy at the moment has been an explicit commitment to the empowerment of service users; that is, the process of giving service users greater choice and control over the services they receive. This can be seen as a countervailing pressure to the issues of accountability described above. However, it is important to consider the mechanism of this process of empowerment and the implications that this might have. Empowerment is perceived as being largely achieved through the application of market mechanisms. This is further discussed in the section on service brokerage. One attempt to provide an overview of the principles underlying the future development of services can be found in 'A new outcomes framework for the assessment of adult social care' produced by the Commission for Social Care Inspection (2006) which in turn is drawn from the White Paper, *Our health, our care, our say* (Department of Health, 2006):

Improved health: enjoying good physical and mental health (including protection from abuse and exploitation). Access to appropriate treatment and support in managing long term conditions independently. There are opportunities for physical activity.
Services promote and facilitate the health and emotional well-being of people who use the services.
Improved quality of life: access to leisure, social activities and life-long learning and to universal, public and commercial services. Security at home, access to transport and confidence in safety outside the home.
Services promote independence, and support people to live a fulfilled life making the most of their capacity and potential.
Making a positive contribution: maintaining involvement in local activities and being involved in policy development and decision-making.
Councils ensure that people who use their services are encouraged to participate fully in their community and that their contribution is valued equally with other people.
Exercise of choice and control: through maximum independence and access to information. Being able to choose and control services and helped to manage risk in personal life.
People who use services, and their carers, have access to choice and control of good quality services, which are responsive to individual needs and preferences.
Freedom from discrimination or harassment: equality of access to services for all who need them.
Those who need social care have equal access to services without hindrance from discrimination or prejudice; people feel safe and are safeguarded from harm.
Economic well-being: access to income and resources sufficient for a good diet, accommodation and participation in family and community life. Ability to meet costs arising from specific individual needs.
People are not disadvantaged financially and have access to economic opportunity and appropriate resources to achieve this.
Personal dignity and respect: not being subject to abuse. Keeping clean and comfortable. Enjoying a clean and orderly environment. There is availability of appropriate personal care.
Adult Social Care provides confidential and secure services, which respects the individual and preserves people's dignity.

Activity

Look at the main headings from the framework for inspecting adult care services above:

- To what extent do you think this framework is likely to lead to the empowerment of people who use care services?
- To what extent do you think it represents a move towards practice based around a social model?
- To what extent is it likely to involve practitioners being either participants in or the objects of surveillance?
- What is needed in order to ensure that the general statements here provide a basis for effective and appropriate practice?

There is a potential tension here between the philosophical position being taken, which is very supportive of the values associated with good practice as outlined in Chapter 5, and the possibility of defensive practice as outlined earlier in this chapter. How this will resolve itself is at this stage unclear.

Diversity, ethnicity and health and social care

There is a long history of people coming to the UK to work in welfare services at all levels, from doctors and qualified nurses through to front line care staff and those who support care. Initially migration was from the Caribbean, later from South Asia and most recently from the former 'Soviet bloc' countries of Eastern Europe. This has major implications for those recruiting health and social care workers, training, the workers themselves and those receiving care. In general terms and with the exception of doctors the care workforce tends to be ethnically diverse at the level of front line practitioners and support staff but increasingly less diverse as we move up through the professional and managerial 'ranks'.

Historically there is also considerable evidence that health and social care services have not been aware of the needs of the whole community and that assumptions have been made on the basis of cultural stereotypes with regard to both care needs and the capacity to provide care. To give one example, assumptions are being made as part of the assessment process about the existence of the extended family that are willing and able to provide care within the Asian community, without this being checked out (see Chapter 9). Furthermore some groups face particular difficulty in gaining any access to services, e.g. the traveller community or some sections of the homeless population.

The reasons for this are many but include direct racism, or other forms of discrimination, the application of stereotypes which influence assessment and what the Macpherson Report (the report into the Metropolitan Police's failed investigation of the killing of Stephen Lawrence) called institutional racism:

> The collective failure of an organisation to provide an appropriate and professional service to people because of their colour, culture or ethnic origin. It can be seen or detected in processes, attitudes and behaviour which amount to discrimination through unwitting prejudice, ignorance, thoughtlessness and racist stereotyping which disadvantages ethnic minority people.
>
> [Racism] persists because of the failure of the organisation openly and adequately to recognise and address its existence and cause by policy, example and leadership. Without recognition and action to eliminate, such racism can prevail as part of the ethos or culture of the organisation. It is a corrosive disease. (Home Office, 1999: 28, para. 6.34)

The concept of institutional racism has been applied to health and social care services in recent years highlighting the impact both on service users in the ways outlined above and in terms of the career progression of workers from minority groups. It remains, though, a difficult and contentious area. Perhaps the most high-profile example in recent years was the case of David 'Rocky' Bennett, an Afro-Caribbean man who was an inpatient at a mental health unit in Norwich and who died after being restrained by staff. The inquiry concluded that institutional racism played a significant part in his death. It is still the case that African and Afro-Caribbean people, especially men, are significantly over-represented in the mental health system as the 2006 'Count me in' Census has identified:

> admission rates were lower than average among the White British, Indian and Chinese groups, and three or more times higher than average in Black and White/Black Mixed groups. In the Other Black group, patients were overall 14 times more likely average to be admitted (amongst men this was almost 18 times – the same as in 2005).

A number of commentators have identified institutional racism as a key factor in this (see for example Pilgrim and Rogers, 2005).

Activity

Some writers have suggested that the way forward is to develop specialised services to meet the needs of particular communities or groups, while others have suggested that the only long-term solution is to ensure that 'mainstream' services are able to meet the needs of the whole community.

o   What do you think are the advantages and disadvantages of each approach?
o   What is the best way forward: is it one or other or both?

Brokerage and markets – choice and consumer culture

In the previous chapter the possible introduction of a form of service brokerage was discussed. This represents a way of 'empowering within the context of a 'mixed economy' approach to the development and delivery of services. It highlights the role of service users as consumers of care services and makes assumptions about both people's willingness and capacity to 'choose' services. There are, though, some very considerable limitations of the model which need to be considered. Hirschman (1970) suggests that there are two fundamental models of empowerment, 'exit' and 'voice'. Exit models work on the assumption that if users do not like a service they will 'exit' this service and use another one. Voice models highlight the limitations of this: that there may not be effective alternatives especially for those who need specialised support, for example. In this model it is not the ability to choose between services but the ability to influence the way in which existing services are delivered that is important. As we move more fully into the mixed economy in both health and social care it becomes increasingly important to think carefully about whether the market/consumer model can provide adequate guarantees in terms of ensuring and protecting the best interests of service users. In this context Hirschman also identifies the significance of a third factor, 'loyalty', which is the tendency of people to accept rather passively whatever is familiar, which again may impact on the consumer model of empowerment. As an example of this we need to think very carefully about whether measured 'satisfaction' of service users through surveys etc. (see Chapter 3) is 'real' or influenced by the factors illustrated above and by the power differentials discussed earlier.

Technology for both workers and users

A further significant issue for the future is the changing role of technology. To give one perhaps controversial example, there are advertisements in the United States from companies which install web cameras and closed-circuit television in the homes of older people so that family members can ensure the safety of 'loved ones'. Once again this raises issues of individual rights versus surveillance and control. While we might wish to accept scrutiny from family members, would it be acceptable if this scrutiny came from the control centre of a care organisation?

Another range of issues stems from the increasing use of IT systems for the storage and transmission of information. Some of the issues are technical ones – to what extent can systems be relied upon to do what they are intended to do? There have been a number of examples in recent years of large-scale IT projects in both the NHS and the wider public sector which have had significant implementation problems. The range of activity for which IT-based systems are expected to be utilised is increasing rapidly, with a range of assessment, recording and control functions being undertaken not just using IT but in an online form. Examples include the Single Assessment Process for Adults, The Common Assessment Framework for Children and Families and the new online Criminal Records Checking System. While there are clearly advantages in terms of facilitating multi-agency working etc. of online and integrated systems, they also raise a number of issues about:

- what information is to be shared and under what circumstances;
- who should have access and how;
- ensuring accuracy and consistency of recording, especially if the same framework is being used by people from different professional backgrounds.

There is therefore a clear need for a range of protocols, which are currently being developed by government. Nonetheless, for many with an interest in this area concerns remain about the difficult balance between civil liberties and the need for the effective monitoring of practice.

In the same way as technology is impacting on the lives of those who work in health and social care, a parallel set of issues is emerging for those who use these services. Technology can in some circumstances be liberating, e.g. through the use of more sophisticated equipment to support people with daily living, or it can be controlling by creating opportunities for increased surveillance and control.

As we reach the end of the book (and as you reach the end of your course) what is the health and social care workforce within which you will be developing your career going to look like? In this book we have already identified a number of key trends:

- The move to a mixed economy of welfare.
- The move to greater emphasis on multi/interprofessional working.
- An increased emphasis on accountability.
- The emergence of a new range of contexts and approaches for working.
- A greater emphasis on supporting service users' rights and choices.

Activity

Looking at this range of issues, what do you see as the main implications for you in terms of your own career development?

Concluding remarks

Crystal ball gazing is of course a slightly dangerous activity; however, there do seem to be a number of ways in which the factors outlined above might influence the future direction of services. In terms of the mixed economy this obviously creates a greater range of potential employers, though there is also some evidence that it has had a negative impact on salaries because of the pressures of competition. The move to greater multi/interprofessional models of working is a more complicated and difficult area to explore, though what is certain is that there will be a need for those working within health and social care to be aware of the changing context and to operate comfortably with a range of other professionals.

Linked to this is the issue of 'deprofessionalisation', the way in which roles formerly carried out by 'professionals' such as nurses, social workers, etc., have increasingly been carried out by other workers, namely health care assistants, social work assistants, etc., leaving professionals to focus on more complex elements of their role. This has been accompanied as discussed previously by an increased element of monitoring of the work of all by external inspectorates. This creates a further set of uncertainties around the boundaries of roles which can be perceived depending upon your viewpoint, such as creating a new, more flexible and possibly creative workforce, or an attempt to devalue professional skills and knowledge. This is a particularly pertinent and positive issue in respect of Foundation Degrees as graduates may well find themselves at the 'cutting edge' with the sorts of skills the new roles are likely to demand, as this debate is played out in the future development of services.

Undeniably the most important set of issues concerns the areas of user empowerment and accountability. As explored previously, there has been a much greater emphasis in recent government policy on the importance of user empowerment, e.g. through the slow introduction of brokerage models or the greater choice being offered to patients around hospital treatment. While it is possible to argue both that progress has been slow and that the model of empowerment has considerable limitations, finding realistic ways of working in genuine partnership with service users is going to be at the heart of the emerging health and social care role. As you develop your career, responding in positive and creative ways to this challenge will be a central element of your effective professional development.

GLOSSARY

This is intended to be a glossary of commonly used health and social care terms which relate to the content of this book.

Abuse – actions which lead to harm to others. This can include physical harm, emotional harm, financial harm or sexual harm. Abuse is usually taken to mean deliberate acts or failures to act; inadvertent harm resulting from a failure to act appropriately is usually referred to as neglect.

Accountability – being responsible for your own actions; this can include accountability to managers, stakeholders and professional bodies (e.g. through codes of conduct).

Acute care – the short-term medical care provided in hospitals (e.g. surgery).

Advocacy – ensuring that those who use care services have a voice. In this context this includes both self-advocacy, which is supporting people in speaking for themselves, and professional advocacy, which is 'speaking up' to ensure users' voices are heard.

Agency – a body providing health and care services; this can be a statutory body (e.g. NHS trust), a private company or a voluntary/charitable organisation. Services can be provided by paid workers or volunteers.

Assessment – the process of identifying an individual's needs (usually taken to mean the formal process of identifying and recording these needs).

Autonomy – the ability of individuals to have their individual rights and choices respected.

Benefits – government-provided financial assistance to help in covering the costs of daily living. They can be 'means tested', i.e. based on an assessment of any other income, and/or eligibility related, i.e. dependent on being in a particular category, e.g. having a particular level of disability.

Care or case management – terms which broadly mean the process of both implementing and managing a care plan.

Care plan – a statement of how needs identified through the assessment process will be met, often involving the collaboration of more than one agency.

Carer – someone who provides substantial support to another person; can be unpaid as an informal carer, e.g. partner, child, friend, or paid as a formal carer.

Case study – a form of research which focuses on a specific individual, agency or event.

Charging – the process of paying for services (see **financial assessment**).

Choice – having the opportunity to select appropriate services, often linked to **consumerism** and the **New Right** critique of services.

Chronic illness – long-standing conditions, often associated with ageing, which cannot be 'cured'.

Commission for Social Care Inspection (CSCI) – the body with responsibility for the inspection of all adult social care services.

Common Assessment Framework – the assessment system used by all agencies working with children designed to support the implementation of 'Every Child Matters'.

Community – a group of people with clearly defined unifying characteristics, e.g. living in the same geographical area or a common culture or ethnicity.

Community care – care provided to enable someone to stay or live within the community.

Confidentiality – the principle that information about individuals is private and should not be inappropriately disclosed.

Consent – the giving of permission for something to happen, e.g. a particular treatment or sharing of information.

Consultation – the active seeking of information or opinion.

Consumerism – the belief that service users in health and social care services should be treated in the same way as customers of other goods and services.

Culture – a shared 'way of life' which might include language, customs, values and patterns of behaviour.

Data – systematically collected information. There are two broad forms: quantitative is the collation of 'factual', often numerical material; qualitative is concerned with perception or opinion.

Demography – the study of the changing characteristics of populations over time in relation to age structure, gender balance, etc.

Direct payments – the system whereby money is given to individuals to enable them to purchase their own care (or care for their children in the case of parents of children with a disability).

Disability – defined by the Disability Discrimination Act 1995 as 'a physical or mental impairment that has a substantial and long-term adverse effect on a person's ability to carry out normal day-to-day activities' (see **medical model** and **social model**).

Discrimination – treating someone less well on the basis of a particular characteristic, e.g. disability or gender.

Diversity – the recognition of the complexity of modern societies and in particular the need to be aware of the importance of culture, religion or language.

Domiciliary care – care within one's own home, also called home care.

Eligibility criteria – criteria defining who is entitled to access to services.

Empowerment – encouraging service users to take as much control as possible over their own lives.

Enabling – working with service users in ways which promote independence.

Ethics – codes giving a moral framework for practice.

Ethnicity – membership of a particular socio-cultural group. Everyone has an ethnicity, as part of either a majority or minority group.

Evaluation – the process of judging whether or not something has been effective.

Evidence-based practice – practice based on the use of research or other evidence.

Fair Access to Care Services – the current government framework of **eligibility criteria** for social care services.

Financial assessment – the process of means testing someone in order to assess their ability to pay for care services.

Formal carer (see **carer**).

General Social Care Council (GSCC) – the body which regulates the social care workforce.

Healthcare Commission – the body with responsibility for regulating health care in both the NHS and private and voluntary sectors.

Home care – an alternative term for **domiciliary care**.

Identity – sense of self; links to a range of other social and cultural factors.

Independence – the ability to control one's own lifestyle.

Independent sector – private and voluntary providers of health and social care services.

Informal carer (see **carer**).

Integrated services – services where workers from different agencies work collaboratively, a form of **multi-agency working**.

Joint working – services where workers from more than one agency work together, again a form of **multi-agency working**.

Key worker – an individual with responsibility for co-ordinating aspects of someone's care.

Learning disabilities/difficulties – an umbrella term for people who have difficulty with some aspect of learning or communication; it covers people with a very wide range of support needs.

Legislation – laws introduced by government which create the legal framework for practice.

Local authority – the elected local level of government which plays a lead role in social care and other related (e.g. education) services.

Medical model – the view that health and disability have a biological or physiological basis and are located within the individual. Intervention should be based on expert assessment and is likely to use intervention through medication or specialist (and sometimes segregated) services.

Mental health – the sense of inner well-being likened to feelings and emotions. In some circumstances difficulties with mental health can be severe requiring short- or longer-term support from a range of services.

Mixed economy – describes the fact that welfare services can or should be provided by a range of public, private and voluntary organisations and funded from a variety of sources such as taxation, charging, etc.

Multi-agency working – an umbrella term for a range of arrangements in which workers work with colleagues from other agencies in a variety of ways (see also integrated services, joint working).

Needs – what a person requires in order to maintain an acceptable quality of life.

Neglect (see **abuse**).

New Labour – the post-1997 Labour Party with its commitment to 'Third Way' politics.

New Right – political approach which emerged in the 1980s with a commitment to reducing the role of government and promoting the role of markets and market-like approaches in health and social care.

NHS – the government-run universal health care system.

Participation – the ability to influence the nature and type of services provided.

Performance indicator – criteria for monitoring the effectiveness of health and social care services.

Primary care – the 'front line' care provided by GPs, dentists, etc.

Primary care trust – the part of the NHS responsible for local services.

Privacy – the right of service users to have individual private space or private conversations.

Private sector – individuals, organisations and companies which provide health and social care services on a 'for-profit' basis.

Protocol – formal rules or guidelines for practice in a particular area.

Provider – an individual or organisation which provides services.

Purchaser – a body which buys health and social care services for either individuals or local populations.

Referral – the process of requesting action or intervention from another agency.

Risk – the possibility that an action or inaction will lead to harm.

Risk assessment – identifying the risks that apply in a particular situation and the likelihood of any of them actually occurring.

Secondary care – care provided in hospital or other referral-based services.

Service user – a person who receives support form health and social care services.

Social model – the view that health and disability are a result of the interplay between individuals and the environment (physical, social and psychological) and that services need to tackle factors such as poverty and social exclusion and public attitudes.

Social policy – the study of welfare-related issues and social and government responses to them.

Social services – social care and related services (e.g. care management and assessment, fostering and adoption) either provided directly or funded through the public sector.

Social Services Department – the local authority department with statutory responsibility for providing or commissioning social care services.

Stakeholder – someone with a direct interest in services, e.g. service users, carers, care staff.

Strategic health authority – the tier of the NHS responsible for strategic planning and co-ordination of services.

Tendering – the process of competitive bidding for contracts to provide services.

Third sector – an umbrella term for non-profit-making organisations, also called the voluntary sector.

User involvement – the process of involving service users in the planning or development of services.

Voluntary sector (see **third sector**).

Volunteer – someone who contributes to the work of organisations without being paid.

Vulnerability – the extent to which someone is 'at risk' (see **risk**).

Welfare services – an umbrella term for the range of services provided for the 'public good', namely health and social care, financial benefits and sometimes education.

Well-being – the sense of being generally healthy, incorporating physical, emotional and spiritual elements as well as adequate command of the resources for living.

Whistleblowing – the decision to disclose poor practice, negligence or illegal acts where these have been covered up by managers within an organisation.

BIBLIOGRAPHY

Abel-Smith, B. (1996) 'The escalation of health care costs: how did we get there?', in *Health Care Reform: The Will to Change*. Paris: OECD, pp. 17–30.

Adams, R. (2003) *Social Work and Empowerment*, 3rd edn. Basingstoke: Palgrave Macmillan.

Adams, R., Dominelli, L. and Payne, M. (2005) 'Transformational social work', in R. Adams, L. Domminelli and M. Payne (eds), *Social Work Futures*. Basingstoke: Palgrave Macmillan.

Ainsworth, M. D. S, Bell, S. M. and Stayton, D. J. (1971) 'Individual differences in strange situation behaviour of one-year olds', in H. R. Schaffer (ed.), *The Origins of Human Social Relations*. London: Academic Press.

Allen, J. (2000) 'Power: its institutional guises (and disguises)', in G. Hughes and R. Fergusson (eds), *Ordering Lives: Family, Work and Welfare*. London: Routledge.

Allott, M. and Robb, M. (eds), (1998) *Understanding Health and Social Care: An Introductory Reader*. London: Sage.

Arber, S. and Cooper, H. (2000) 'Gender inequalities in health across the life course', in E. Annandale and K. Hunt (eds), *Gender Inequalities in Health*. Buckingham: Open University Press.

Arber, S. and Thomas, H. (2001) 'From women's health to a gender analysis of health', in W. Cockerham (ed.), *The Blackwell Companion to Medical Sociology*. Oxford: Blackwell, pp. 94–113.

Aspis, S. (1997) 'Self-advocacy for people with learning difficulties: does it have a future?', *Disability and Society*, 12: 647–54. (Also in Bytheway, B., Bacigalupo, V., Bornat, J., Johnson, J. and Spurr, S. (eds) (2002) *Understanding Care, Welfare and Community*. London: Open University/Routledge.)

Aspis, S. (1999) 'What they don't tell disabled people with learning difficulties', in M. Corker and S. French (eds), *Disability Discourse*. Buckingham: Open University Press.

Baggott, R. (2004) *Health and Health Care in Britain*, 3rd edn. Basingstoke: Palgrave Macmillan.

Bagihole, B. (1997) *Equal Opportunities and Social Policy*. London: Longman.

Bandura, A., Ross, D. and Ross, S. A. (1961) 'Transmission of aggression through observation of aggressive models', *Journal of Abnormal and Social Psychology*, 63: 575–82.

Banks, S. (2000) *Ethics and Values in Social Work*, 2nd edn. Basingstoke: Palgrave.

Banks, S. (2006) *Ethics and Values in Social Work*, 3rd edn. Basingstoke: Palgrave.

Beauchamp, T. and Childress, J. (2001) *Principles of biomedical ethics*. Oxford: Oxford University Press.

Becker, M. H. and Rosenstock, I. M. (1984) 'Compliance with medical advice', in A. Steptoe and A. Mathews (eds), *Health Care and Human Behaviour*. London: Academic Press.

Beckett, C. and Maynard, A. (2005) *Values and Ethics in Social Work: An Introduction.* London: Sage.

Bell, J. (2005) *Doing your research project: a guide for first-time researchers in education,* 4th edn. Buckingham: Open University Press.

Beresford, P. and Croft, S. (2003) 'Involving service users in management: citizenship, access and support', in J. Reynolds et al. (eds), *The Managing Care Reader.* London: Routledge/OU.

Blaxter, M. (2004) *Health.* Cambridge: Polity Press.

Boud, D., Keogh, R. and Walker, D. (1985) 'Promoting reflection in learning', in R. Edwards, A. Hanson and P. Raggatt (eds) (1996), *Boundaries of Adult Learning.* London: Routledge/OU.

Bowlby, J. (1969) *Attachment and Loss,* Vol. 1. New York: Basic Books.

Bradshaw, J. (1972) 'A taxonomy of social need', in G. Mclachlan (1972), *Problems and Progress in Medical Care.* Oxford: Nuffield Foundation.

Brechin, A. (2000) 'Introducing critical practice', in A. Brechin, H. Brown and M. Eby (eds), *Critical Practice in Health and Social Care.* London: Sage/OU.

Bronfenbrenner, U. (1979) 'Contexts of child rearing: problems and prospects', *American Psychologist,* 34: 844–50.

Brown, G. and Harris, T. (1978) *The Social Origins of Depression.* London: Tavistock.

Brown, H. and Walmsley, J. (1997) 'When "Ordinary" isn't enough', in J. Bornat et al. (eds), *Community Care: A Reader,* 2nd edn. London: Sage/OU.

Burton, G. and Dimbleby, R. (1988) *Between Ourselves: An Introduction to Interpersonal Communication.* London: Edward Arnold.

Bury, M. R. (1982) 'Chronic illness as biographical disruption', *Sociology of Health and Illness,* 4: 167–82.

Busfield, J. (2006), 'Pills, power, people: sociological understandings of the pharmaceutical industry', *Sociology,* 40(2): 297–314.

Carr-Hill, R. (1987) 'The inequalities in health debate: a critical review of the issues', *Journal of Social Policy,* 16(4): 509–42.

Centre for Evidence Based Social Services (2004) www.ripfa.org.uk/archive

Charmaz, K. (1999) 'Experiencing chronic illness', in Albrecht et al. (2003) *The Handbook of Social Studies in Health and Medicine.* Thousand Oaks, CA: Sage.

Cochrane, A. L. (1972) *Effectiveness and Efficiency: Random Reflections on Health Services.* Leeds: Nuffield Provincial Hospital Trust.

Cottrell, S. (2003) *Skills for Success.* Basingstoke: Palgrave Macmillan.

CSCI (2006) Support Brokerage: A discussion paper, available at http://www.csci. org.uk/about_us/publications/support_brokerage.aspx.

Davies, M. (1981) *The Essential Social Worker: A guide to positive practice.* London: Heinemann Educational Books.

Dawson, A. and Butler, I. (2003) 'The morally active manager', in J. Henderson and D. Atkinson (eds) (2004), *Managing Care in Context.* London: OU/Routledge.

Deurcombe, M. (2003) *The Good Reserch Guide,* 2nd edn. Maidenhead: Open University Press.

Department for Education and Skills (2001) *Special Educational Needs Codes of Practice.* London: TSO.

Department for Education and Skills (2006) *Working Together to Safeguard Children.* London: TSO.

Department for Education and Skills (2006) *Care Matters: Transforming the Lives of Children and Young People in Care*. London: TSO.

Department of Health (2000) *No Secrets: guidance on developing and implementing multi-agency policies and procedures to protect vulnerable adults from abuse*. London: HMSO.

Department of Health (2001) *Valuing People: A New Strategy for Learning Disability for the 21st Century*. London: TSO.

Department of Health (2003a) *Fair access to care services – guidance on eligibility criteria for adult social care*. London: Department of Health.

Department of Health (2003b) *The Victoria Climbie Inquiry: A report by Lord Laming*. London: HMSO.

Department of Health (2005) *Case management competences framework for the care of people with long term conditions*. London: Deptartment of Health.

Department of Health (2005) *Independence, Well-being and Choice: our vision for the future of social care for adults in England*, Cm6499. London: Department of Health.

Department of Health (2006) *Our health, our care, our say: a new direction for community services White Paper*, Cm6737. London: Department of Health.

Dickens, C. (1896) *Dombey and Son*. London: Chapman and Hall.

Doyal, L. and Gough, I. (1991) *A Theory of Human Need*. London: Palgrave Macmillan.

Eby, M. (1994) 'Competing values', in V. Tschudin (ed.), *Ethics: Conflicts of Interest*. London: Scutari Press.

Eby, M. (2000a) 'Understanding professional development', in A. Brechin, H. Brown and M. Eby (eds), *Critical Practice in Health and Social Care*. London: Sage/OU.

Eby, M. (2000b) 'The challenge of values and ethics in practice', in A. Brechin, H. Brown and M. Eby (eds), *Critical Practice in Health and Social Care*. London: Sage/OU.

Erikson, E. H. (1963) *Childhood and Society*, 2nd edn. New York: Norton Penguin Books, Hogarth Press.

Gallie, D., White, M., Cheng, Y. and Tomlinson, M. (2001) 'The restructuring of work since the 1980s', in N. Abercrombie and A. Warde (eds), *The Contemporary British Society Reader*. Cambridge: Polity Press.

Giddens, A. (1991) *Modernity and Self-Identity. Self and Society in the Late Modern Age*. Cambridge: Polity Press.

Giddens, A. (2000) *The Third Way and its critics*. London: Polity Press.

Gimlin, D. (2002) *Body Work: Beauty and Self-Image in American Culture*. Berkeley, CA: University of California Press.

Goffman, E. (1963) *Stigma: Notes on the Management of Spoiled Identity*. New York. Prentice Hall.

Gomm, R. (1993) 'Issues of power in health and welfare', in J. Walmsley, J. Reynolds, P. Shakespeare and R. Woolfe (eds) (1993) *Health, Welfare and Practice: Reflecting on Roles and Relationships*. London: Sage.

Gomm, R. and Davies, C. (eds) (2000) *Using Evidence in Health and Social Care*. London: Sage.

Goodley, D. (2004) 'Who is disabled? Exploring the scope of the social model of disability', in J. Swain et al. (eds), *Disabling Barriers – Enabling Environments*, 2nd edn. London: Sage/OU.

Goodley, D. and Ramcharan, P. (2005) 'Advocacy, campaigning and people with learning difficulties', in G. Grant et al. (eds), *Learning Disability: A life cycle approach to valuing people*. Maidenhead: Open University Press/McGraw-Hill Education.

Hall, E. T. (1966) *The Hidden Dimension*. New York: Garden City.

Hartley, P. (1993) *Interpersonal Communication*. London: Routledge.

Hirschman, A. (1970) *Exit, Voice, and Loyalty: Responses to Decline in Firms, Organizations, and States*. Boston: Harvard University Press.

HM Treasury (2006) *Budget details 2006–2008*. London: HMSO.

Hochschild, A. R. (1983) *The Managed Heart: Commercialization of Human Feeling*. Berkeley, CA: University of California Press.

Home Office (1999) *The Stephen Lawrence inquiry; Report of an inquiry by Sir William Macpherson of Cluny*. London: The Stationery Office.

Hugman, R. (2003) 'Professional values and ethics in social work: reconsidering post-modernism', *British Journal of Social Work*, 33: 1025–41.

Hurd, G. (ed.) (1974) *Human Societies*. London: Routledge.

Husband, C. (1995) 'The morally active practitioner and the ethics of anti-racist social work', in R. Hugman and D. Smith (eds), *Ethical Issues in Social Work*. London: Routledge.

Illich, I. (1976) *Limits to Medicine*. London: Marion Boyars.

Inskipp F. (1996) *Skills Training for Counselling*. London: Sage.

Johnson, D. and Johnson, F. (1998) *Joining Together: Group Theory and Group Skills*. London: Prentice Hall.

Katbamna, S., Bhakta, P., Ahmad, W., Baker, R. and Parker, G. (2002) 'Supporting South Asian carers and those they care for: the role of the primary health care team', *British Journal of General Practice*, 52(477): 300–5.

Kobasa, S. C. (1979) 'Stressful life events, personality and health: an inquiry into hardiness', *Journal of Personality and Social Psychology*, 65: 207.

Kobus, K. (2003) 'Peers and adolescent smoking', *Addiction*, 98: 37–55.

Kübler-Ross, E. (1969) *On Death and Dying*. London: Tavistock.

Lazarus, R. S. and Folkman, S. (1984) *Stress: Appraisal and coping*. New York: Springer.

Lewis, S., Saulnier, M. and Renaud, M. (2000) 'Reconfiguring health policy: simple truths, complex solutions', in G. L. Albrecht, R. Fitzpatrick and S. C. Scrimshaw (eds), *The Handbook of Social Studies in Health & Medicine*. London: Sage.

Link, B. and Phelan, J. (1995) 'Social conditions as fundamental causes of disease', *Journal of Health and Social Behavior*, extra issue: 80–94.

Magnani, L. E. (1990) 'Hardiness, self-perceived health, and activity among independently functioning older adults', *Scholarly Enquiry for Nursing Practice*, 4(3): 171–84.

Martin, V. and Henderson, E. (2001) *Managing in Health and Social Care*. London: OU/Routledge.

Maslow, A. (1970) *Motivation and Personality*. New York: Harper and Row.

McBeath, G. and Webb, S. A. (2002) 'Virtue ethics and social work: being lucky, realistic, and not doing one's duty', *British Journal of Social Work*, 32: 1015–36.

McKeown, T. (1976) *The Modern Rise of Population*. London: Edward Arnold.

Mears, R. (1992) 'Debating health inequalities', in M. O'Donnell (ed.), *Introductory Readings in Sociology*. Walton-on-Thames: Nelson.

Nettleton, S. (2006) *The Sociology of Health and Illness*, 2nd edn. Cambridge: Polity Press.

Nelson-Jones, R. (1997) *Practical Counselling and Helping Skills*, 4th edn. London: Continuum.

Nussbaum, M. (2000) *Women and human development: The capabilities approach*. New York: Cambridge University Press.

O'Donnell, M. (1987) *A New Introduction to Sociology*. Walton-on-Thames: Nelson.

Oliver, M. (1981) 'The individual model of disability', in V. Finkelstein (ed.) (1983), *Rehabilitation: Supplementary Readings*. P556 Rehabilitation: A collaborative approach to work with disabled people, Milton Keynes: Open University Press.

Open University (1996) *Speaking Out for Equal Rights*, Workbook 2, K503 Working as Equal People. Milton Keynes: Open University Press.

Pahl, J. (1990) 'Household spending, personal spending and the control of money in marriage', *Sociology*, 24(1): 119–38.

Papadopoulos, R. (2003) 'The Papadopoulos, Tilki and Taylor model for the development of cultural competence in nursing', *Journal of Health, Social and Environmental Issues*, 4: (1).

Payne, M. (1997) *Modern Social Work Theory*, 2nd edn. Basingstoke: Macmillan.

Payne, S. (2006) *The Health of Men and Women*. Cambridge: Polity Press.

Pearce, S. and Reynolds, J. (2003) in J. Henderson and D. Atkinson (eds), *Managing Care in Context*. London: Routledge/OU.

Pilgrim, D. and Rogers, A. (2005) *A Sociology of Mental Health and Illness*. Maidenhead: Open University Press.

Putnam, R. (2000) *Bowling Alone: The collapse and revival of American community*. New York: Simon and Schuster.

Quinn, F. M. (1988) 'Reflection and reflective practice', in C. Davies, L. Finlay and A. Bullman (eds), *Changing Practice in Health and Social Care*, London: Sage/OU.

Raphael, D. D. (1994) *Moral Philosophy*, 2nd edn. Oxford: Oxford University Press.

Robson, C. (2002) *Real World Research*. London: Blackwell.

Rogers, C. R. (1951) *Client Centred Therapy*. London: Constable.

Russell, G. (2000) *Essential psychology for nurses and other health professionals*. London: Routledge.

Rutter, M. (1972) *Maternal Deprivation Reassessed*. Harmondsworth: Penguin Education.

Scambler, G. (2003) *Sociology as Applied to Medicine*. Oxford: Elsevier.

Scambler, G. (2004) 'Reframing stigma: felt and enacted stigma and challenges to the sociology of chronic and disabling conditions', *Social Theory and Health*, 2: 29–46.

Schön D. A. (1983) *The Reflective Practitioner: How Professionals Think in Action*. London: Basic Books.

Scott, R. A. (1969) *The making of blind men*. New York: Sage Foundation.

Scott, R. A. (1970) 'The construction of conceptions of stigma by professional experts', in D. Boswell and J. Wingrove (eds) (1974), *The Handicapped Person in the Community*. London: Tavistock/OU.

Scourfield, P. (2005) 'Understanding why Carers Assessments do not always take place', *Practice*, 17(1): 15–30.

Seligman, P. (1975) *Helplessness: On Depression, Development and Death*. San Francisco: Freeman.

Shannon, C. E. and Weaver, W. (1949) *The Mathematical Theory of Communication*. Urbana, IL: University of Illinois Press.

Shardlow, S. (2002) 'Values, ethics and social work', in R., Adams, L. Dominelli and M. Payne (eds), *Social Work Theories, Issues and Critical Debates*, 2nd edn. Basingstoke: Palgrave/OU.

Skills for Health (2005) www.skillsforhealth.org.uk [accessed April 2006].

Smith, M. K. (1996/2001) 'Action research', *the encyclopedia of informal education, www.infed.org/research/b-actres.htm* (accessed January 2005).

Stewart, W. (1992) *An A–Z of Counselling Theory and Practice.* London: Chapman and Hall.

Swain, J., Finkelstein, V., French, S. and Oliver, M. (eds) (1993) *Disabling Barriers – Enabling Environments.* London: Sage/OU.

Swain, J., Gillman, M. and French, S. (1998) *Confronting Disabling Barriers: Towards making organisations accessible.* Birmingham: Venture Press.

Swain, J., French, S., Barnes, C. and Thomas, C. (2004) *Disabling Barriers – Enabling Environments,* 2nd edn. London: Sage/OU.

Tajfel, H. and Fraser, C. (eds) (1978) *Introducing Social Psychology.* Harmondsworth: Penguin.

Terrisse, B. (2000) 'The resilient child: theoretical perspectives and a review of the literature', in R. Croker (ed.), *PCERA 2000 Children and Youth at Risk: The symposium report.* Ottawa: Canadian Education Statistics Council.

Thomas, C. (1993) 'Deconstructing concepts of care', *Sociology,* 27(4): 649–69.

Thompson, N. (1995) *Theory and Practice in Health and Social Welfare.* Milton Keynes: Open University Press.

Thompson, N. (2006) *Anti-Discriminatory Practice,* 4th edn. Basingstoke: Palgrave.

Thompson, N. (2003) *Promoting Equality: Challenging Discrimination and Oppression in the Human Services,* 2nd edn. London: Macmillan.

Turner, B. (1995) *Medical Power and Social Knowledge.* London: Sage.

Twigg, J. and Atkin, K. (1994) *Carers Perceived: Policy and Practice in Informal Care.* Buckingham: Open University Press.

White, C., Wiggins, R., Blane, D., Whitworth, A. and Glickman, M. (2005) 'Person, place or time? The effect of individual circumstances, area and changes over time on mortality in men, 1995–2001', *Health Statistics Quarterly,* 28: Winter.

Wilkinson, R. (2000) *Mind the Gap: Hierarchies, Health and Human Evolution.* London: Weidenfeld & Nicolson.

Wolfensberger, W. (1998) *A brief introduction to Social Role Valorisation: A high-order concept for addressing the plight of societally devalued people, and for structuring human services,* 3rd edn. Syracuse, NY: Training Institute for Human Service Planning, Leadership & Change Agentry.

Wolfensberger, W. and Tullman, S. (1982) 'The principle of normalization', in B. Bytheway et al. (eds) (2002), *Understanding Care, Welfare and Community.* London: OU/Routledge.

INDEX